Operative Techniques in Gynecologic Surgery

Urogynecology

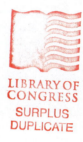

Operative Techniques in Gynecologic Surgery

Urogynecology

Series Editor

Jonathan S. Berek, MD, MMS

Laurie Kraus Lacob Professor
Stanford University School of Medicine
Director, Stanford Women's Cancer Center
Senior Scientific Advisor, Stanford Cancer Institute
Director, Stanford Health Communication Initiative
Advancing Communication Excellence at Stanford
Stanford, California

Christopher M. Tarnay, MD

Clinical Professor
Division Chief, Female Pelvic Medicine and Reconstructive Surgery
Departments of Obstetrics & Gynecology and Urology
David Geffen School of Medicine at UCLA
Los Angeles, California

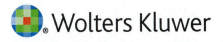

Philadelphia • Baltimore • New York • London
Buenos Aires • Hong Kong • Sydney • Tokyo

Executive Editor: Rebecca Gaertner
Acquisitions Editor: Chis Teja
Product Development Editor: Ashley Fischer
Editorial Assistant: Brian Convery
Marketing Manager: Rachel Mante Leung
Production Project Manager: David Saltzberg
Design Coordinator: Teresa Mallon
Artist/Illustrator: Jason M. McAlexander, MPS North America LLC
Manufacturing Coordinator: Beth Welsh
Prepress Vendor: Aptara, Inc.

Copyright © 2019 Wolters Kluwer.

All rights reserved. This book is protected by copyright. No part of this book may be reproduced or transmitted in any form or by any means, including as photocopies or scanned-in or other electronic copies, or utilized by any information storage and retrieval system without written permission from the copyright owner, except for brief quotations embodied in critical articles and reviews. Materials appearing in this book prepared by individuals as part of their official duties as U.S. government employees are not covered by the above-mentioned copyright. To request permission, please contact Wolters Kluwer at Two Commerce Square, 2001 Market Street, Philadelphia, PA 19103, via email at permissions@lww.com, or via our website at lww.com (products and services).

9 8 7 6 5 4 3 2 1

Printed in China

Library of Congress Cataloging-in-Publication Data

Names: Tarnay, Christopher M., editor.
Title: Operative techniques in gynecologic surgery. Urogynecology / [edited by] Christopher M. Tarnay.
Other titles: Urogynecology
Description: Philadelphia : Wolters Kluwer, [2019] | Includes bibliographical references and index.
Identifiers: LCCN 2018018109 | ISBN 9781496321060 (hardback : alk. paper)
Subjects: | MESH: Pelvic Floor Disorders–surgery | Urogenital Surgical Procedures | Gynecologic Surgical Procedures
Classification: LCC RD571 | NLM WP 155 | DDC 617.4/6059–dc23
LC record available at https://lccn.loc.gov/2018018109

This work is provided "as is," and the publisher disclaims any and all warranties, express or implied, including any warranties as to accuracy, comprehensiveness, or currency of the content of this work.

This work is no substitute for individual patient assessment based upon healthcare professionals' examination of each patient and consideration of, among other things, age, weight, gender, current or prior medical conditions, medication history, laboratory data and other factors unique to the patient. The publisher does not provide medical advice or guidance and this work is merely a reference tool. Healthcare professionals, and not the publisher, are solely responsible for the use of this work including all medical judgments and for any resulting diagnosis and treatments.

Given continuous, rapid advances in medical science and health information, independent professional verification of medical diagnoses, indications, appropriate pharmaceutical selections and dosages, and treatment options should be made and healthcare professionals should consult a variety of sources. When prescribing medication, healthcare professionals are advised to consult the product information sheet (the manufacturer's package insert) accompanying each drug to verify, among other things, conditions of use, warnings and side effects and identify any changes in dosage schedule or contraindications, particularly if the medication to be administered is new, infrequently used or has a narrow therapeutic range. To the maximum extent permitted under applicable law, no responsibility is assumed by the publisher for any injury and/or damage to persons or property, as a matter of products liability, negligence law or otherwise, or from any reference to or use by any person of this work.

LWW.com

To Matthew and MaiAnh, continue to be curious and kind.
To my wife LanAnh, there is no better sage.

Contributing Authors

Morgan E. Fullerton, MD
Female Pelvic Medicine and Reconstructive Surgery Fellow
Department of Obstetrics and Gynecology
David Geffen School of Medicine at UCLA
Los Angeles, California

Erin M. Mellano, MD
Assistant Clinical Professor of Obstetrics and Gynecology
Division of Female Pelvic Medicine and Reconstructive Surgery
David Geffen School of Medicine at UCLA
Los Angeles, California

Lisa Rogo-Gupta, MD, FACOG FPMRS
Assistant Clinical Professor of Obstetrics and Gynecology
  (and, by courtesy, Urology)
Stanford University School of Medicine
Director, Ambulatory Gynecology and Gynecologic Specialties
Stanford, California

Contributing Authors

Foreword

Operative Techniques in Gynecologic Surgery is presented in four volumes—*Gynecology, Reproductive Endocrinology and Infertility, Urogynecology*, and *Gynecologic Oncology*. Their purpose is to provide clear and concise illustrations of essential operations representing the fundamental procedures for each of these subspecialties.

This series is distinct from other textbooks in gynecology because of their focus as an illustrated practical guide to the surgical processes using easily accessible photographs and video clips.

In *Gynecology*, the first in this series, we depict the most common operations of our clinical specialty. The second does the same for *Reproductive Endocrinology and Infertility*, the third for *Urogynecology and Pelvic Reconstructive Surgery*, and the fourth for *Gynecologic Oncology*. We assembled a group of outstanding authors and contributors to produce these volumes, under the guidance of highly regarded expert senior book editors.

Gynecology—Tommaso Falcone, MD, is the Head of Gynecology at the Cleveland Clinic and is well known for his expertise in the operative management of benign gynecologic conditions. He and his co-authors, M. Jean Uy-Kroh, MD, and Linda D. Bradley, MD, have carefully assembled a very useful series of photographs and videos that highlight the fundamentals of the surgical operations in our field.

Reproductive Endocrinology and Infertility—Steven Nakajima, MD, is a Clinical Professor of Obstetrics and Gynecology in the Fertility and Reproductive Health Group, Stanford University School of Medicine, and his focus is on the procedural and operative aspects of reproductive medicine. Along with the contributions from his colleagues, Travis W. McCoy, MD, and Miriam S. Krause, MD, this book will serve as a clear summary of the necessary procedures in this specialty.

Urogynecology—Christopher M. Tarnay, MD, is an Associate Professor at the David Geffen School of Medicine at UCLA, where he is the Chief of Urogynecology and Reconstructive Pelvic Surgery. He and his colleague, Lisa Rogo-Gupta, MD, Clinical Assistant Professor, Stanford University School of Medicine, have contributed substantially to our understanding of the important discipline of Female Pelvic Medicine and Reconstructive Surgery.

Gynecologic Oncology—Kenneth D. Hatch, MD, is a well-known gynecologic oncologist who is a Professor at the University of Arizona School of Medicine. He is considered one of the primary experts in the surgical management of gynecologic malignancies. Dr. Hatch and his contributors will provide a precise visual explanation of the essential operative treatments in this subspecialty.

We intend this series to enhance the educational activities for our colleagues in the practice of Gynecology and dedicate this series to our patients in the hope that it will facilitate optimal care and improved outcomes.

Jonathan S. Berek, MD, MMS
Series Editor, *Operative Techniques in Gynecologic Surgery*
Laurie Kraus Lacob Professor
Stanford University School of Medicine
Director, Stanford Women's Cancer Center
Senior Scientific Advisor, Stanford Cancer Institute
Director, Stanford Health Communication Initiative
Advancing Communication Excellence at Stanford
Stanford, California

Preface

This volume is the distillation of close to two decades of efforts to improve. The authors and I share these efforts in the form of experiences passed on by our mentors, from our colleagues, and through the years of self-exploration as we have striven toward the elusive goal of mastery. At its roots, early innovative urogynecologic procedures essentially helped define the emerging discipline of surgical gynecology in the early 19th century. For over a hundred years practitioners caring for women with prolapse and incontinence have struggled to find durable solutions to these most common and at times the most debilitating medical and social afflictions. The field of Urogynecology (now Female Pelvic Medicine and Reconstructive Surgery) was fundamentally established to try to understand how to do things better.

My view of contemporary Urogynecology is shaped by a unifying paradigm. Modern medicine is epitomized by the creation of subspecialization and niche practice. Through this lens it is understandable or even logical that the female pelvis was quite literally divided among three separate disciplines: Urology (anterior compartment), Gynecology (middle compartment), and Colorectal/General Surgery (posterior compartment). As a urogynecologist and now "Female Pelvic Medicine Specialist," those borders can be erased. The crossover of bladder, vaginal, and anorectal conditions not only share anatomic physical boundaries but also very often share a pathophysiology. These pelvic floor conditions can only be adequately addressed with a thorough understanding and acceptance of holistic nature that these three compartments frequently exist as a manifestation of one system.

The purpose of this volume is to detail a practical yet thoughtful approach to the surgical management of pelvic floor disorders. Current urogynecology is minimally invasive surgery at its core. The procedures and techniques outlined will focus on the innovations that preserve this tenant. For practical purposes we break surgical techniques by compartment, recognizing the interdependency of concomitant procedures to address multi-compartment problems. We present the established traditional approaches with a nod toward innovation with graft augmentation and application of robotics.

This effort was truly a collaborative one. Co-authors Dr. Lisa Rogo-Gupta and Dr. Erin M. Mellano, are two of the most gifted reconstructive surgeons, brightest minds and more importantly most thoughtful and compassionate physicians I have had privilege with which to work. I want to acknowledge contributor Dr. Morgan E. Fullerton, a current fellow and next generation leader in FPMRS, for her contributions to the text and her dedication to the field.

Christopher M. Tarnay, MD

Contents

Chapter 1   **Anterior Vaginal Wall Repair**   1
Lisa Rogo-Gupta and Christopher M. Tarnay

Chapter 2   **Apical Prolapse Repair: Vaginal Approach**   17
Christopher M. Tarnay

Chapter 3   **Posterior Vaginal Wall Repair**   31
Erin M. Mellano and Lisa Rogo-Gupta

Chapter 4   **Apical Prolapse Repair: Abdominal Approach**   49
Christopher M. Tarnay

Chapter 5   **Urinary Incontinence Procedures**   65
Lisa Rogo-Gupta and Christopher M. Tarnay

Chapter 6   **Genitourinary Fistula**   97
Erin M. Mellano and Lisa Rogo-Gupta

Chapter 7   **Rectovaginal Fistula and Perineal Lacerations**   123
Erin M. Mellano

Chapter 8   **Approach to Removal of Vaginal Mesh**   141
Lisa Rogo-Gupta

Chapter 9   **Urethral Diverticulum and Anterior Vaginal Wall Cysts**   155
Christopher M. Tarnay and Morgan E. Fullerton

Chapter 10   **Cystoscopy**   173
Lisa Rogo-Gupta

Index   181

Chapter 1
Anterior Vaginal Wall Repair

Lisa Rogo-Gupta, Christopher M. Tarnay

GENERAL PRINCIPLES
IMAGING AND OTHER DIAGNOSTICS
PREOPERATIVE PLANNING
SURGICAL MANAGEMENT
PROCEDURES AND TECHNIQUES
    Traditional Midline Repair
    Graft-Augmented Repair
    Paravaginal Repair
PEARLS AND PITFALLS
POSTOPERATIVE CARE
OUTCOMES
COMPLICATIONS

Anterior Vaginal Wall Repair
Lisa Rogo-Gupta, Christopher M. Tarnay

GENERAL PRINCIPLES

Definition

- Pelvic organ prolapse (POP) is descent of the vaginal wall and associated organs. There are two methods of classifying POP:
  - By prolapsed organ:
    - Urethrocele (urethra)
    - Cystocele (bladder)
    - Uterus/cervix (uterine/cervical)
    - Vaginal cuff (post-hysterectomy)
    - Small intestine (enterocele)
    - Rectum (rectocele)
    - Perineum (perineocele)
  - By compartment:
    - Anterior (may include urethra and/or bladder)
    - Apical (may include uterus/cervix, post-hysterectomy vagina, or small intestine)
    - Posterior (may include small intestine, rectum, and/or perineum)
- While it is estimated that 50% of asymptomatic women have mild POP, only 3% of adult women report POP symptoms.[1]
- Women with a history of one vaginal delivery are four times more likely to have surgery for POP compared to women who have not, while women who have a history of two vaginal deliveries are eight times more likely. Approximately 1 in 1,000 adult women undergoes POP surgery annually.

History

- A patient presenting with POP most commonly reports a feeling of vaginal bulging, pelvic pressure, generalized heaviness, or backache.[2] Symptoms typically have an insidious onset over a period of months to years, culminating in an acute event such as the visualization of a vaginal mass or difficulty with the general function of affected organ(s). POP is worsened with prolonged standing, activity, straining, and position change, and often improved by laying supine.
- Patient with anterior vaginal wall (AVW) prolapse may present with associated symptoms such as:
  - POP symptoms
    - Vaginal bleeding, discharge, or infection
    - Need for vaginal digitation of the prolapsing organ
  - Voiding symptoms
    - Dysuria
    - Hesitancy
    - Slow, intermittent, or change in stream
    - Feeling of incomplete bladder emptying requiring straining, position change, or digital replacement of the POP
    - Need to immediately void again
  - Urinary incontinence (see Chapter 5)

Physical Examination

- General pelvic examination (see Table 1.1).
- Demonstration of POP on examination involves visualization of vaginal wall descent with strain with physical exertion (see Fig. 1.1; Video 1.1). This is standardly

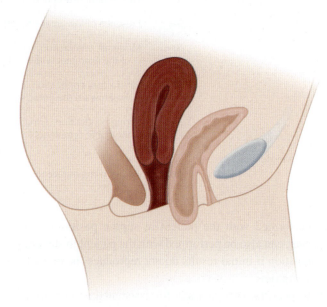

Figure 1.1. Anterior vaginal prolapse (cystocele) extending beyond the hymen.

Table 1.1 Physical Examination of Urogynecologic Patients

Organ System	Examination Findings
General	Signs of systemic illness Peripheral edema
Skin	Ecchymosis, ulcerations, rashes, changes in pigmentation
Gynecologic	External female genitalia Vulva (labial architecture, skin lesions, signs of atrophy) Glands (Skene, Bartholin) Urethral meatus Vaginal wall appearance (scarring, ulcers, lesions) Cervix and uterus (appearance, size, mobility, masses, tenderness) Adnexa (mobility, masses, tenderness) Rectum (anal tone, rectovaginal septum)
Neurologic	Sensory evaluation (if indicated)
Musculoskeletal	Mobility, ambulation, strength
Additional	Post-void residual Urinalysis Bladder diary (or "voiding log")
Pelvic organ prolapse	Anterior, apical, and posterior compartments Relax and strain positions
Urethral hypermobility	Urethral mobility during Valsalva Hypermobility defined as ≥30 degrees
Urinary incontinence	Involuntary leakage during Valsalva or cough
Pelvic floor evaluation	Tenderness, strength Perineal body and levator ani
	0 — Lack of muscle response
	1 — Flicker of nonsustained contraction
	2 — Presence of low-intensity, but sustained, contraction
	3 — Moderate contraction, felt like an increase in intravaginal pressure, which compresses the fingers of the examiner with small cranial elevation of the vaginal wall
	4 — Satisfactory contraction, compressing the fingers of the examiner with elevation of the vaginal wall toward the pubic symphysis
	5 — Strong contraction, firm compression of the examiner's fingers with positive movement toward the pubic symphysis
Fistula evaluation	Tampon test Imaging studies using intravenous or intrarectal contrast

performed with the patient in supine position, however, can also be performed with the patient in standing position if initial results do not reproduce the patient's symptoms.
- Inspect the vaginal walls for associated abnormalities (bleeding, discharge, or infection).
- Perform bimanual examinations to assess for pelvic masses and pelvic organ mobility.
- In cases where urinary incontinence is present, further evaluation may be undertaken (see Chapter 5).

Differential Diagnosis
- The differential diagnosis of AVW prolapse includes:
  - Vaginal wall masses
    - Inclusion cyst (see Fig. 1.2)
    - Leiomyoma
    - Vaginal septum
    - Urethral diverticula (Fig. 1.3)
    - Skene duct cyst or abscess
    - Gartner duct
    - Ectopic ureter

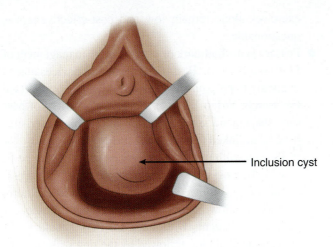

Figure 1.2. Patient presenting with vaginal bulging, found to have vaginal wall inclusion cyst.

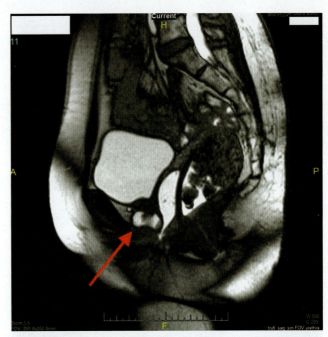

Figure 1.3. Urethral diverticulum (red arrow). Sagital view magnetic resonance imaging.

- Hydrocele of the canal of Nuck
- Malignancy
- Compression by extrinsic factors
  - Pelvic or intra-abdominal mass
  - Ascites or hemoperitoneum
- Foreign body (see Fig. 1.4)

Nonoperative Management

- Behavior and lifestyle modifications are considered first-line management for AVW defects and prolapse in general. These include addressing factors impacting chronic increases in intra-abdominal pressure including weight loss, chronic cough, constipation, and repetitive heavy lifting. Factors impacting tissue quality should also be addressed such as tobacco use, chronic steroids, and hypoestrogenic state.

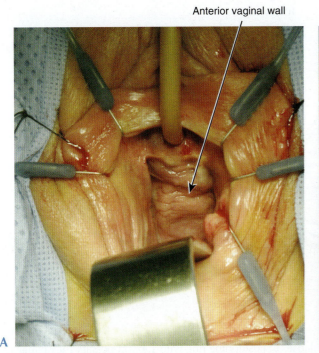
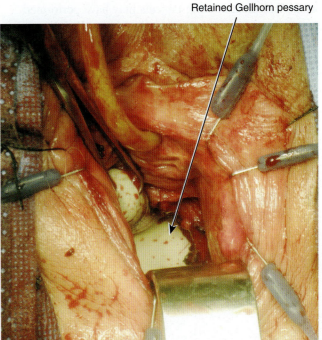

Figure 1.4. A, B: Patient presenting with pelvic pressure and heaviness, found to have vaginal foreign body (pessary) behind the anterior vaginal wall.

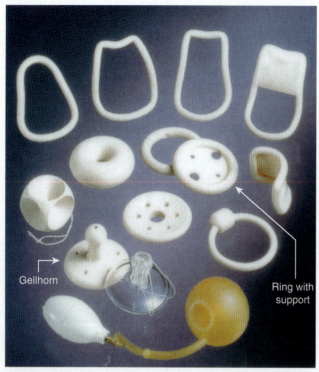

Figure 1.5. Example of different pessary types. (From Ricci SS. *Essentials of Maternity, Newborn, and Women's Health Nursing*. 3rd ed. Philadelphia, PA: Wolters Kluwer; 2012.)

- Exacerbating factors should be controlled. These may include physical activity or heavy lifting. Modification of exercise, work, or personal responsibilities may be required.
- Pelvic floor physical therapy has equivocal efficacy in the treatment of POP. Patients may have performed pelvic floor exercise in the past (known as "Kegel exercises") but are often unable to achieve or even assess proper performance. For prolapse, effectiveness of exercises alone remain low and cost-effectiveness is questionable.
- Pessary is the hallmark of nonoperative management of POP (see Fig. 1.5).[3] Pessaries are support devices placed vaginally to prop up and replace prolapsing organs (see Fig. 1.6A,B; Video 1.2). There are a variety of pessary shapes and sizes; however certain characteristics have been linked to successful fitting.
  - Patients with mild to even advanced POP may be fit with the ring-style support pessary, and if unsuccessful can be followed by attempts with the Gellhorn. There is a low likelihood of success with subsequent fittings.[4] Patients with stage IV POP should be fit with the Gellhorn, followed by the ring with support, for a success rate is 64% and 36%, respectively.
  - Factors associated with difficult pessary fitting:
    - Prior POP repair
    - Prior hysterectomy
    - Short total vaginal length (less than 6 cm)
    - Wide genital hiatus (greater than 4 cm)

IMAGING AND OTHER DIAGNOSTICS

- Diagnostic evaluation may be used when additional information might impact patient counseling and treatment planning. For example, in cases where initial history and examination are inconsistent or inconclusive and a clear diagnosis is not obtained (see Fig. 1.7).
- Further diagnostics are not required when treating patients with uncomplicated POP.
- Diagnostic evaluation may include one or more of the following:
  - Ultrasound, computerized tomography.
  - Dynamic magnetic resonance imaging for POP (see Fig. 1.8).[5,6]

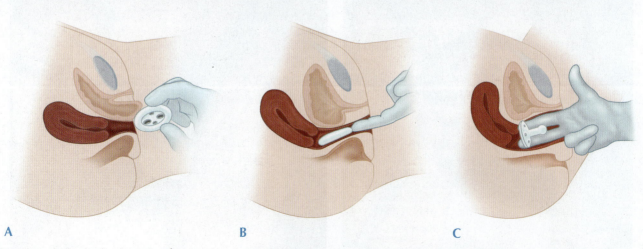

Figure 1.6. **A:** Beginning insertion for anterior or apical vaginal prolapse. **B:** Positioning ring with support pessary for vaginal prolapse. **C:** Fitting a Gellhorn pessary.

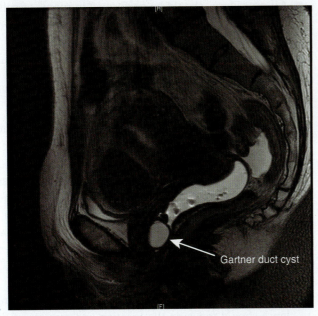
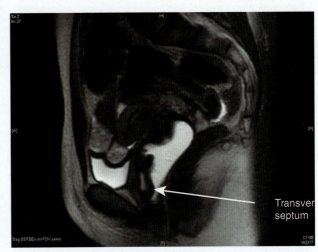

Figure 1.7. **A:** Gartner duct cyst diagnosed by MRI. **B:** Transverse vaginal septum diagnosed by MRI.

- Evaluation related to associated urinary symptoms of AVW prolapse.
  - Post-void residual (PVR) is the measurement of urine in the bladder following urination by transabdominal ultrasound or by catheterization. PVR assessment should be performed when patients report urinary symptoms as listed above.
  - Urinalysis or culture should be performed to exclude urinary tract infection in patients reporting urinary symptoms suggestive of infection.
  - Severe AVW prolapse has been associated with hydronephrosis in 5% of women necessitating surgery. However, given the majority of women are asymptomatic and possess normal renal function, preoperative screening is not required.[7]

PREOPERATIVE PLANNING

- The fundamental goal of all prolapse treatment is to improve quality of life. Preoperative planning begins with an overall assessment of the patient's reported symptoms, objective findings, and most importantly, treatment goals. Understanding of risks, benefits, and treatment alternatives as well as physical capacity to manage unexpected outcomes is essential.
- For patients desiring surgical correction, consider:
  - Documenting discussion of or attempts at nonsurgical management such as behavior modification, pelvic floor exercises, and pessary use prior to surgical management.
  - Consideration of age, activity level, and need for possible repeat treatment when considering the type of surgical treatment options.
  - Physical ability to use indwelling or clean intermittent catheters in cases of postoperative urinary retention.

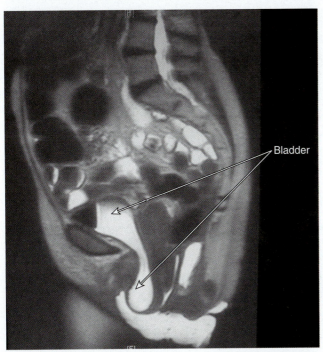

Figure 1.8. Anterior vaginal wall prolapse demonstrated on dynamic MRI. Contrast is placed in the bladder, vagina, and rectum, and MRI is obtained while the patient is asked to strain.

- Informed consent regarding the safety and efficacy of any material used for augmenting the repair including possible short- and long-term complications.
- Traditional midline plication should be considered in these scenarios:
  - Central AVW prolapse
  - Primary AVW repair
- Paravaginal repair should be considered in these scenarios:
  - Lateral AVW prolapse
  - Primary AVW repair
- Graft-augmented repair should be considered in these scenarios:
  - Recurrent AVW prolapse
  - Absent or deficient host endopelvic fascia
  - High risk for recurrence: high physical demand

SURGICAL MANAGEMENT

- There are several methods for surgical management for AVW prolapse. Perioperative risks are generally low similar to other benign gynecologic surgery, and most procedures can be performed with either general or regional anesthesia.
- All procedures should be performed in rooms of sufficient size to allow for the surgeon and assistant as well as cystoscopy equipment.
- Urinary infection should be ruled out and PVR should be considered prior to AVW repair procedures.

Positioning

- AVW repair is performed with the patient in lithotomy position similar to other vaginal or perineal procedures.
  - Various lithotomy stirrups are available to assure patient safety and comfort, minimizing risk for related injury (litho image Chapter 5, see Fig. 5.6).
  - Arms may be left untucked for easy intravenous access by the anesthesiologist or nurse if needed.

Approach

- The approach to surgical management of AVW prolapse should focus on the location and severity of the prolapse. Women who have AVW prolapse are likely to have a component of apical prolapse (see Chapter 2) which will impact surgical outcomes if not concomitantly addressed. Women who undergo isolated AVW repair have a higher reoperation rate compared to those who undergo concurrent apical repair (20% vs. 11%).[8]

Traditional Midline Repair

- Traditional midline repair, also referred to as anterior colporrhaphy, involves plicating the fibromuscular layer of the AVW in the midline. The bladder is thereby supported by the inward imbricated tissue, and the vaginal epithelium is closed over the repair (see Tech Fig. 1.1).

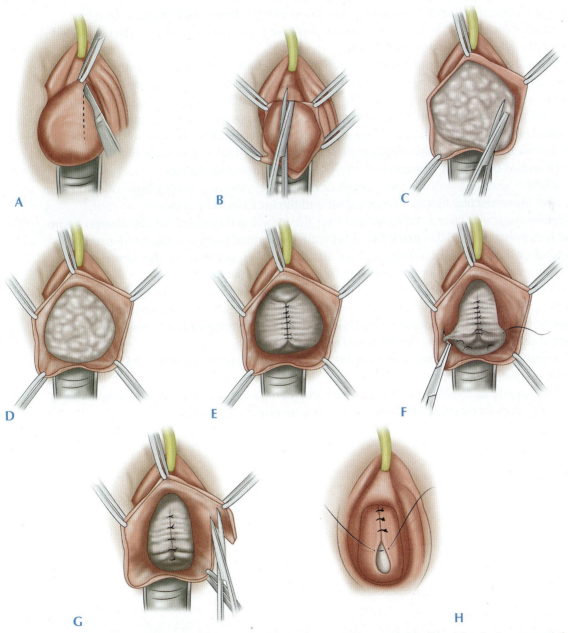

Tech Figure 1.1. Classic anterior colporrhaphy. **A:** Initial midline anterior vaginal wall incision is demonstrated. **B:** The midline incision is extended using scissors. **C:** Sharp dissection of the bladder off the vaginal wall should be lateral to the superior pubic ramus, and the base of the bladder should be dissected off the vaginal cuff or cervix to the level of the preperitoneal space of the anterior cul-de-sac. **D:** The bladder has been completely mobilized off the vagina. **E:** Initial plication layer is placed. **F:** Second plication layer is placed, which commonly requires further mobilization of vaginal muscularis off of the vaginal epithelium. The most proximal stitch involves plication of the inside of the vaginal wall at the level of the vaginal apex or upper portion of the cervix. **G:** The completed second plication layer and the trimming of excess vaginal mucosa are demonstrated. **H:** Closure of vaginal mucosa is demonstrated. (Adapted from Karram MM. *Surgical Management of Pelvic Organ Prolapse.* Philadelphia, PA: Elsevier/Saunders; 2013.)

- A catheter should be placed into the bladder to maintain drainage throughout the procedure.
- Utilization of a Scott style self-retaining retractor is a vital tool to facilitate all vaginal surgery.
- The vaginal epithelium is mobilized laterally and the AVW prolapse is identified. The distal portion is typically at the level of the bladder neck (see **Pearls and Pitfalls**), and the more proximal is typically the most dependent portion of the prolapse.
- Local anesthetic with a vasoconstrictor agent (epinephrine or Pitressin) can be injected beneath the epithelium. Injection is often used to hydrodissect the proper tissue plane and facilitate entry. Commonly used preparations include bupivacaine 0.25% with or without epinephrine, dilute vasopressin, and normal saline 0.9%.
- A single vertical incision in the vaginal wall is made (see **Pearls and Pitfalls**). An initial horizontal incision at the point of maximal prolapse may also be used and then extended vertically after dissection of epithelium.
- Using a sharp, narrow-tipped scissors such as Metzenbaums, the vaginal epithelium is dissected off the underlying tissues starting at the cut edge and travelling proximally and laterally. Countertraction is provided by the surgical assistant using forceps. Dissection is continued until the entire AVW prolapse has been exposed. This is repeated on the contralateral side. Dissection should be carried all the way out to the inferior pubic ramus.
  - *Traditional midline repair*: depth of dissection is superficial. A thin layer of epithelium is dissected off and the fibromuscular layer left intact over the bladder.
  - *Midline graft-augmented repair*: depth of dissection is deeper. A thick layer of epithelium and fibromuscular tissue is dissected off and the intact bladder remains.
- The fibromuscular layer is then plicated over the imbricated bladder. An absorbable suture such as polyglactin 910 is used. This is typically performed using a series of interrupted sutures or figure-of-eight technique. Care should be taken not to place the sutures too deeply as to avoid bladder transgression or ureteral obstruction.
- Wide lateral support can be achieved with a second supporting layer using absorbable suture. Placing a suture through the lateral aspect of dissection into perivesical fascia at border of inferior pubic ramus on both sides. Two to three additional sutures are placed in dorsal progression. Sutures are then tied down sequentially.
- Diagnostic cystoscopy should be performed to evaluate bladder integrity and to confirm bilateral ureteral efflux.
- Excess vaginal epithelium may be trimmed and then closed over the midline repair. This is typically performed using an absorbable suture in a running fashion.

Graft-Augmented Repair

- Grafts may be added to traditional midline repair in an effort to improve durability when host endopelvic fascia is absent or deficient (see Outcomes section below) (see Tech Fig. 1.2). The most commonly used materials are nonabsorbable synthetic grafts, however autografts and absorbable allografts and xenografts are also available.
- Steps are performed as for traditional repair detailed above with the following exceptions:
    - Depth of epithelial dissection is deeper when synthetic grafts are used. A thick layer of epithelium and fibromuscular tissue is dissected off and the intact bladder remains. This is to ensure adequate epithelial coverage over the graft and decrease the risk of graft exposure.
    - The graft is secured in place laterally after completion of the midline repair.
    - Redundant vaginal epithelium should be preserved and minimally trimmed when utilizing grafts.
    - The skin incisions are closed with care not to incorporate the graft material into the closure.

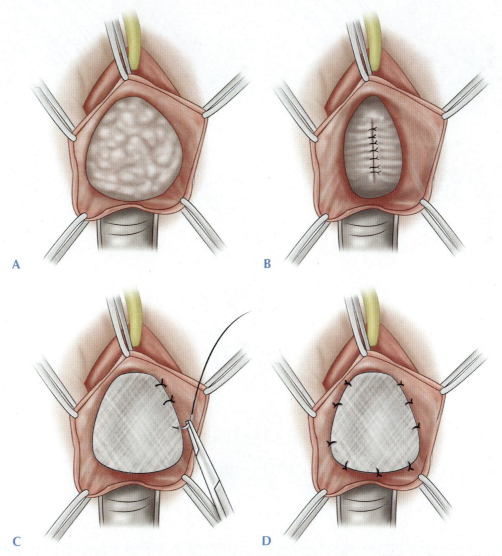

Tech Figure 1.2. Anterior vaginal repair with graft. **A:** The bladder is dissected bilaterally and off the vaginal apex. **B:** Midline plication is completed. **C:** Absorbable sutures are placed at lateral most aspect of dissection incorporating pervesical fascia under epithelium at border of inferior pubic rami bilaterally. **D:** The graft is attached bilaterally, and all sutures are tied, supporting the bladder. (Adapted from Karram MM. *Surgical Management of Pelvic Organ Prolapse*. Philadelphia, PA: Elsevier/Saunders; 2013.)

Paravaginal Repair

- Paravaginal repair may be performed when lateral defects in the AVW support are noted. This can be identified by the lack of presence of the lateral sulci in the anterior vaginal wall (AVW). This represents detachment of the lateral vagina from the arcus tendineus fascia pelvis (ATFP). These defects can occur unilaterally or bilaterally. Paravaginal defects can be identified clinically by using a long instrument to reduce the vaginal bulge along the lateral sulcus margin parallel to the ischial spine. If the AVW defect is resolved, this supports the presence of a paravaginal detachment. If the vaginal bulge persists, then a central or midline defect is suspected.

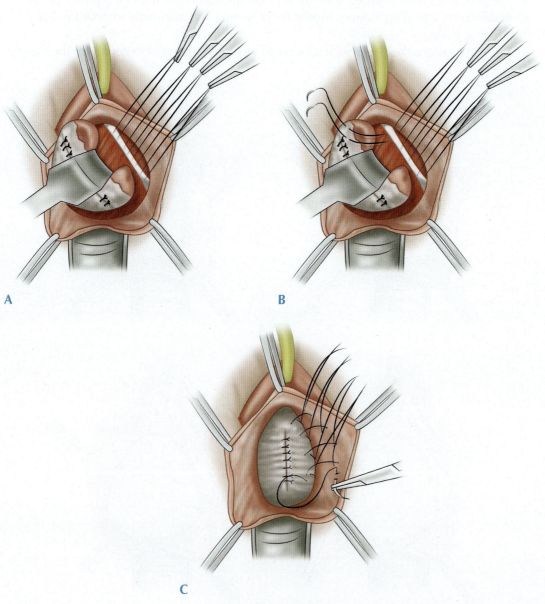

Tech Figure 1.3. Surgical steps for vaginal paravaginal (3-point) repair. **A:** Three to four sutures are passed through the ATFP overlying the fascia over the levator ani muscle (point 1). **B:** Each suture is passed through the lateral edge of the detached endopelvic fascia (point 2). **C:** Each suture is passed through the full thickness of the vaginal wall excluding the epithelium (point 3). (Adapted from Karram MM. *Surgical Management of Pelvic Organ Prolapse*. Philadelphia, PA: Elsevier/Saunders; 2013.)

- Initial steps are performed as for traditional repair detailed above with the following alterations:
    - Lateral dissection is carried further out to the ATFP or "white line." This requires dissection and then perforation through the levators to access the paravaginal space. The paravaginal space is contiguous with the space of Retzius. The ATFP extends from the ischial spine to the posterior inferior aspect of the symphysis pubis and is located proximal to the obturator internus.
    - To facilitate suture placement a Capio (Boston Scientific, Marlborough, MA) device may be used. Sutures are placed through the white line near the level of the ischial spine and another two sutures spaced 2 to 3 cm apart heading toward the pubic bone. The sutures are then ipsilaterally affixed to the endopelvic fascia over the bladder at the corresponding level. This is repeated on the contralateral side if bilateral defects are present. The sutures are tied down to elevate the AVW and restore continuity of the vaginal lateral support (see Tech Fig. 1.3).
    - The repair can also be performed using an abdominal approach, whereby sutures are similarly placed to repair the fascial detachment (see Tech Fig. 1.4). This approach requires a vaginal finger to elevate the vaginal fibromuscular layer into the surgical field.

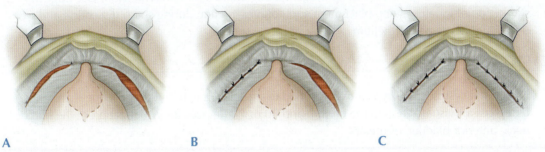

A B C

Tech Figure 1.4. Abdominal paravaginal defect repair reattaches the pubocervical fascia to the white lines bilaterally. **A:** A patient with bilateral paravaginal defects. The repair has been started on the left with sutures at the two extremes of the defect. **B:** The repair is complete on the left side. **C:** Both sides are repaired. (Adapted from Shull BL. How I do abdominal paravaginal repair. *J Pelvic Surg*. 1995;1:43.)

PEARLS AND PITFALLS

ANTERIOR VAGINAL WALL (AVW) LANDMARKS

- ○ Apply gentle traction on an inflated Foley catheter to bring the balloon to a comfortable position in the bladder neck. Palpation on the vaginal side will identify the location of the bladder neck. Measurement from the bladder neck to the proximal aspect of the prolapse can be marked for assistance with incision planning.

BLADDER DISSECTION

- ✗ During access into paravaginal space avoid bladder injury by staying right on or "hugging" the posterior aspect of pubic ramus during penetration with curved scissor.

ANTERIOR VAGINAL WALL REPAIR

- ○ Suture placement during wide lateral AVW repair is facilitated by placing non-dominant finger behind vaginal epithelium to help gauge depth and adequate placement in perivesical fascia.
- ○ To find correct avascular plane and avoid bladder injury during anterior vaginal dissection create a 2–3 mm edge of vaginal epithelium along entire after initial incision. Use edge as starting point for allis clamp placement and counter traction during sharp dissection and undermining vaginal epithelium.

CYSTOSCOPY

- ○ Diagnostic cystoscopy is typically performed using a 17-French rigid cystoscope. Lens angle is 0 degrees for visualization of the urethra and 30 or 70 degrees for visualization of the bladder neck, anterior bladder, or ureters.

POSTOPERATIVE CARE

- Postoperative care following urogynecologic procedures is similar to that for other benign gynecologic surgery.
- Antibiotics are *recommended* for the following procedures:
  - Vaginal surgery: Guidelines from the surgical care improvement project (SCIP) recommend using a first- or second-generation cephalosporin for 24 hours.
- Continuous bladder drainage is *not required* for the following procedures:
  - POP surgery: Overall risk of urinary retention is low and does not justify continuous drainage in all patients. The decision should be made on a case-by-case basis and patients should be counseled on the risks and benefits of multiple options. Patients at high risk for postoperative retention may remain with an indwelling catheter or be instructed on self-catheterization to decrease anxiety and to avoid visits to emergency facilities.
- Physical activity restriction is *recommended* for the following procedures:
  - POP surgery, vaginal surgery: Sexual activity and aerobic exercise should be limited in the immediate postoperative period.
- Follow-up evaluation is *recommended* for the following procedures:
  - Approximately 2 weeks for patients at high risk of urinary retention following cystoscopic procedures.
  - Approximately 4 to 6 weeks in low-risk patients following vaginal surgery.

OUTCOMES

- *Traditional midline repair*
  - Reported success rates vary widely depending on definition used, ranging from 39%, if defined as POP-Q stage 0 or I, to 88% if defined as no prolapse beyond the hymen and asymptomatic and not retreated.[9]
- *Traditional midline versus graft-augmented repair (synthetic)*

- Multicenter, randomized, controlled trial comparing the two methods demonstrates traditional repair outcomes of approximately 60% subjective and 35% objective success rate, and low reoperation rate of less than 1% at 1 year.[10] This compared to repairs augmented with synthetic nonabsorbable grafts which demonstrated approximately 75% subjective and 60% objective success rate, and a 3% reoperation risk for exposure at 1 year with synthetic nonabsorbable grafts.
- Others describe risk of erosion of synthetic grafts may be as high as 11% to 15% in the first year[11] with a reoperation rate of 7%.[12]
- Systematic reviews demonstrate synthetic grafts (absorbable and nonabsorbable) all improve objective outcomes compared to traditional midline repair alone. Synthetic graft use is associated with higher blood loss, operative time, occurrence of other POP, and de novo Stress Urinary Incontinence (SUI) compared to native tissue repair.
- *Traditional midline versus graft-augmented repair (biologic)*
  - Systematic reviews demonstrate improved objective outcomes with graft augmentation but no significant difference in subjective outcomes or quality of life.[12]
- *Traditional midline versus graft-augmented (synthetic) versus paravaginal repair (biologic)*
  - No significant difference in overall failure (defined as bulge symptoms and at least stage III AVW prolapse), however objective failure was statistically significant for the different methods (defined as stage III AVW prolapse) and occurred in 58%, 18%, and 46%, respectively.[13]
  - Synthetic graft use was associated with 14% erosion rate.

COMPLICATIONS

- Traditional midline repair carries a 1% to 3% risk of bladder injury, de novo SUI, infection, or pain.
- Graft-augmented repair carries a 12% risk of de novo SUI, and 1% to 4% risk of bladder injury, hemorrhage, infection, or pain. Synthetic grafts have an 11% to 15% erosion/complication risk.

KEY REFERENCES

1. Wu JM, Vaughan CP, Goode PS, et al. Prevalence and trends of symptomatic pelvic floor disorders in U.S. women. *Obstet Gynecol.* 2014;123(1):141–148.
2. Haylen BT, de Ridder D, Freeman RM, et al. An International Urogynecological Association (IUGA)/International Continence Society (ICS) joint report on the terminology for female pelvic floor dysfunction. *Neurourol Urodyn.* 2010;29(1):4–20.
3. Culligan PJ. Nonsurgical management of pelvic organ prolapse. *Obstet Gynecol.* 2012;119(4):852–860.
4. Cundiff GW, Amundsen CL, Bent AE, et al. The PESSRI study: symptom relief outcomes of a randomized crossover trial of the ring and Gellhorn pessaries. *Am J Obstet Gynecol.* 2007;196(4):405 e401–e408.
5. Gousse AE, Barbaric ZL, Safir MH, Madjar S, Marumoto AK, Raz S. Dynamic half Fourier acquisition, single shot turbo spin-echo magnetic resonance imaging for evaluating the female pelvis. *J Urol.* 2000;164(5):1606–1613.
6. Comiter CV, Vasavada SP, Barbaric ZL, Gousse AE, Raz S. Grading pelvic prolapse and pelvic floor relaxation using dynamic magnetic resonance imaging. *Urology.* 1999;54(3):454–457.
7. Costantini E, Lazzeri M, Mearini L, Zucchi A, Del Zingaro M, Porena M. Hydronephrosis and pelvic organ prolapse. *Urology.* 2009;73(2):263–267.
8. Eilber KS, Alperin M, Khan A, et al. Outcomes of vaginal prolapse surgery among female Medicare beneficiaries: the role of apical support. *Obstet Gynecol.* 2013;122(5):981–987.
9. Chmielewski L, Walters MD, Weber AM, Barber MD. Reanalysis of a randomized trial of 3 techniques of anterior colporrhaphy using clinically relevant definitions of success. *Am J Obstet Gynecol.* 2011;205(1):69 e61–e68.
10. Altman D, Vayrynen T, Engh ME, Axelsen S, Falconer C; Nordic Transvaginal Mesh Group. Anterior colporrhaphy versus transvaginal mesh for pelvic-organ prolapse. *N Engl J Med.* 2011;364(19):1826–1836.
11. Sokol AI, Iglesia CB, Kudish BI, et al. One-year objective and functional outcomes of a randomized clinical trial of vaginal mesh for prolapse. *Am J Obstet Gynecol.* 2012;206(1):86 e81–e89.
12. Maher CM, Feiner B, Baessler K, Glazener CM. Surgical management of pelvic organ prolapse in women: the updated summary version Cochrane review. *Int Urogynecol J.* 2011;22(11):1445–1457.
13. Menefee SA, Dyer KY, Lukacz ES, Simsiman AJ, Luber KM, Nguyen JN. Colporrhaphy compared with mesh or graft-reinforced vaginal paravaginal repair for anterior vaginal wall prolapse: a randomized controlled trial. *Obstet Gynecol.* 2011;118(6):1337–1344.

Chapter 2
Apical Prolapse Repair: Vaginal Approach

Christopher M. Tarnay

GENERAL PRINCIPLES
IMAGING AND OTHER DIAGNOSTICS
PREOPERATIVE PLANNING
SURGICAL MANAGEMENT
PROCEDURES AND TECHNIQUES
   Uterosacral Ligament Vault Suspension
   Sacrospinous Ligament Vault Suspension
   Uterosacral Ligament Hysteropexy
PEARLS AND PITFALLS
POSTOPERATIVE CARE
OUTCOMES
COMPLICATIONS

Apical Prolapse Repair: Vaginal Approach

Christopher M. Tarnay

GENERAL PRINCIPLES

Definition

- Prolapse of the vaginal apex occurs when there are deficiencies in support of the upper portion of the vagina. The primary support structures involved are the uterosacral ligament and cardinal ligament complex. These have been described as level I support by DeLancey. Disruption or weakness of level I support during childbirth, trauma, or gynecologic surgery is considered to be the cause of apical prolapse (Fig. 2.1). There are a number of terms that have been used to describe apical prolapse. When the uterus is in place: uterine prolapse, uterocervical prolapse, and procidentia. When the uterus is removed: vault prolapse, cuff prolapse, enterocele, and apical prolapse are all described. Identification of apical defects is in general more difficult than other types of prolapse. This is because significant laxity of the apical vaginal support can exist but still visually remain above the vaginal opening. This is an important clinical consideration as the apex of the vagina is closely associated with the support of other vaginal compartments. Most relevantly the apex and the anterior wall are codependent and it is uncommon to have anterior vaginal laxity without concomitant apical descent. The surgical approach and correction of apical support remain a challenge for many surgeons.

Differential Diagnosis

- Anterior or posterior vaginal prolapse
- Vaginal wall cysts

Nonoperative Management

- Most forms of prolapse can be managed with nonsurgical therapy in the form of a pessary. Current quality guidelines encourage all patients be offered pessary management prior to surgical therapy. Pessaries are intravaginal support devices and are designed to either "prop up" the vagina by using the bony and musculature architecture to function as a lever (Fig. 2.2) or to occupy the vaginal canal as a "space-occupying" device (Fig. 2.3) to prevent prolapse. Contemporary pessaries are made of silicone although the fundamental concept and even design have remained relatively unchanged over the years. Pessaries are first-line treatment options. Although pessaries may ultimately not be a suitable long-term solution, they should be offered to all patients with symptoms prior to considering surgical treatment. Women with wide genital hiatus or short vaginal length have higher rates of unsuccessful pessary use and at risk for pessary expulsion.

IMAGING AND OTHER DIAGNOSTICS

- A thorough and thoughtful physical exam of the pelvis and vaginal canal under strain is usually the only necessary tool a surgeon requires. Vaginal and pelvic exam

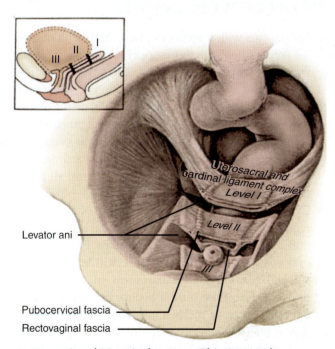

Figure 2.1. Level I is apical support. This proximal suspension includes the uterosacral ligament and cardinal ligament complex. Level II shows the lateral attachment to the arcustendineus fascia of the pelvis. Level III shows the lateral attachment and anterior attachment of connective tissue to the lateral arcustendineus fascia and posterior pubic symphysis. (Adapted from DeLancey JO. Anatomic aspects of vaginal eversion after hysterectomy. *Am J Obstet Gynecol.* 1992;166:1717–1724.)

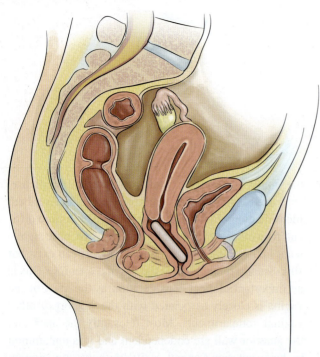

Figure 2.2. Ring pessary for prolapse. (From Jones HW, Rock JA, eds. *Te Linde's Operative Gynecology*. 11th ed. Philadelphia, PA: Wolters Kluwer; 2015.)

reliably identify all clinically relevant vaginal compartment prolapse. For post-hysterectomy prolapse, identifying the herniating visceral structures (high rectocele vs. enterocele or an anterior enterocele) may sometimes be warranted. In this setting, augmenting a physical exam with imaging can be additive.

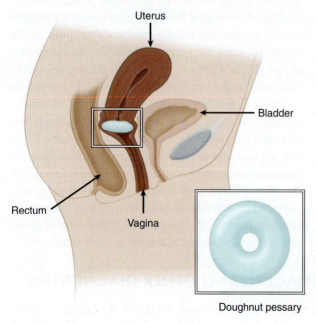

Figure 2.3. Donut pessary for prolapse.

- Ultrasound can be used to characterize pelvic floor musculature, internal genital anatomy, and pelvic organ support. Ultrasound is very technique dependent but may identify the involved compartment of prolapse. Intravaginal and transperineal sonography have been utilized to identify vaginal support defects. Use of ultrasound can also be utilized to evaluate levator ani anatomy and the relationship to the pelvic sidewall.
- Magnetic resonance imaging (MRI): Dynamic MRI with the patient straining can accurately identify the prolapsing structures and also provide useful information about involved organs such as uterus, ovaries, bladder, and rectum. Utilizing the bony pelvis landmarks, the severity of the prolapse can be measured, and MR images provide an illustrative picture of the severity of the condition.
- Imaging is most useful when a careful physical examination cannot definitively isolate the prolapsing structures. Post-hysterectomy posterior prolapse is particularly challenging to identify proximal posterior defects from apical defects representing small bowel herniation such as an enterocele.

PREOPERATIVE PLANNING

- For patients with a uterus in place, discussion of uterine preservation with hysteropexy versus hysterectomy with vault suspension is critical. The reflexive position for prolapse management has traditionally been uterine removal despite no evidence that the uterus plays a meaningful role in the etiology of genital prolapse. For women who are not family complete it is prudent to delay surgical correction until after childbearing, as is the case for surgical management for almost all pelvic floor disorders.
- Cystoscopic evaluation at the time of surgery is required to ensure bladder integrity and ureteral function after vaginal reparative procedures. Preprocedural cystoscopy is not required as it will rarely impact surgical planning or management in women with prolapse. Exceptions are a history of previous suburethral surgery or mesh implantation where urethral and/or bladder integrity is in question. Preprocedural oral phenazopyridine or perioperative (intravenous dye using indigo carmine, methylene blue, or sodium fluorescein) is indispensable for ureteral efflux visualization.
- Bowel preparation is not considered essential and with enhanced recovery protocols is not recommended due to concerns related to dehydration and electrolyte

imbalance. However, bowel preparation or enemas may be implemented to reduce rectal and sigmoid contents particularly when in patients with large posterior defects and stool pocketing or in patients with defecatory dysfunction.

SURGICAL MANAGEMENT

- Prolapse is a condition impacting quality of life. It is imperative that patients understand that prolapse, even advanced prolapse, need not be treated if symptoms are not bothersome nor limiting activity or function. Further, one must delineate symptoms related to prolapse as opposed to symptoms that may not be directly related to the prolapse. For example, bladder overactivity and urinary urge incontinence may not be meaningfully improved with prolapse correction. Similarly, back pain, suprapubic pressure, or constipation may also be independent of vaginal prolapse.
- Once surgery is decided, a route of approach needs to be determined. It is rare that a minimally invasive approach to prolapse cannot be performed.

Positioning

- The most common position for all vaginal reparative surgery is dorsal lithotomy. There are many options for leg support. In the author's experience, all reconstructive procedures can be accomplished with the use of "yellowfin" style stirrups. With these stirrups, the foot, lower leg, and calf are supported with equal distribution of pressure. One needs to avoid "high" lithotomy position which is extension of the knee greater than 90 degrees or hyperflexion of the hip. Proper positioning can minimize the risk of peripheral neuropathy arising from excessive hip flexion, abduction, and external hip rotation that can occur with other types of supports (Fig. 2.4).
- Other aspects are to ensure patient is sufficiently positioned at the "break" of the operative table. Having the perineum at or just below the break of the table ensures proper exposure and will reduce the limitations for posterior vaginal retraction or instrument contact with the table.

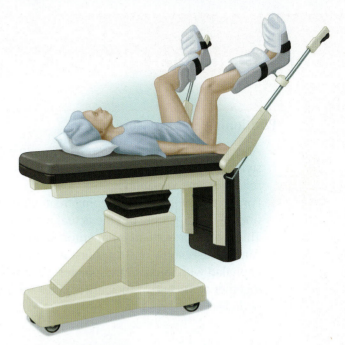

Figure 2.4. Lithotomy.

Approach

- With the benefits of shorter hospitalization, reduced postprocedural pain requirements, and quicker convalescence, a minimally invasive surgery (MIS) approach is preferred for any type of reparative procedure for prolapse. An acceptable approach is in the form of a vaginal or laparoscopic surgery. There are few instances when an MIS approach is not feasible. Vaginal or laparoscopic approaches can be done within 24-hour hospitalizations. Both have similar postprocedural restrictions. Both have roughly equivalent convalescence and postoperative pain medication requirements. In this chapter we will focus on vaginal approach only.

Vaginal Approach

The critical feature when utilizing a vaginal route for apical prolapse is to select an identifiable and adequate support structure within the pelvis with which to affix the vaginal vault. Though several techniques have been described for the correction of apical prolapse, the two most utilized and well-studied employ fixation to either the uterosacral ligaments or to the sacrospinous ligaments.

Uterosacral Ligament Vault Suspension

Positioning and Exposure

- After proper positioning, ensure adequate exposure with the use of a self-retaining Scott style retractor. In our practice we prefer the Lone Star retractor system (Trumbull, CT) for its reliability and versatility.
- For women who are undergoing treatment for uterine prolapse the critical intervention is not the hysterectomy but the actual management of the apex after the uterus is removed. This is true for both an intraperitoneal or extraperitoneal approach.
- After hysterectomy one must first ensure all pedicles are hemostatic and pack the bowel cephalad with laparotomy sponges. We prefer pediatric laparotomy sponges (two tied together at the tail) as they are smaller and less likely to abrade or disrupt the hysterectomy pedicles (Tech Fig. 2.1).

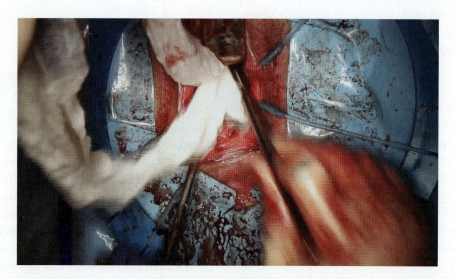

Tech Figure 2.1. Pack bowels with pediatric laparotomy sponges.

Identifying and Suturing the Uterosacral Ligament

- Starting on the patient's right, use Heaney retractors placed at the 10 and 4 o'clock position to expose the posterior peritoneum (Tech Fig. 2.2).
- The posterior vaginal cuff is ipsilaterally grasped with Allis clamps and placed on traction.
- The middle finger of the surgeon's nondominant hand is placed in the rectum and with upward palpation toward the peritoneum the uterosacral ligament can be then identified (Tech Fig. 2.3). This should produce the tactile sensation of a thick "guitar string" and will be readily discernible even in the most lax of prolapse. The only way the ligament can be reliably located is with rectal palpation with concomitant vaginal traction as the ligament is very difficult to palpate transperitoneally alone.

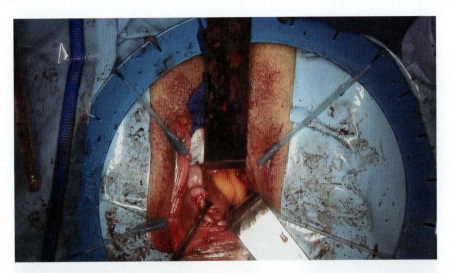

Tech Figure 2.2. Retract at 9:00 and 4:00 for right side.

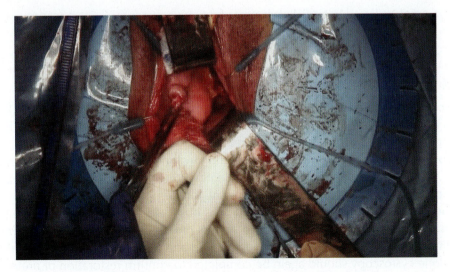

Tech Figure 2.3. Rectal examination to identify and palpate uterosacral ligament.

- Visualization can be facilitated with the use of lighted retractors or with surgeon's headlamp.
- A 2.0 monofilament, permanent or delayed absorbable suture, such as polypropylene or polydioxanone sulfate, is placed lateral to medial through the ligament (Tech Fig. 2.4). The first suture should be placed at the level of the ischial spine. This is normal anatomic position of the cervicovaginal junction and a sensible location for the cuff's new resting position.
- A second suture of the same can then be placed 1 cm more cephalad than the previous. Both sutures are tagged and secured to the retractor frame with the needles still intact until time for fixation to the vaginal cuff.
- For identification, by convention, the more cephalad suture can be tagged with a curved hemostat and the caudal suture with a straight hemostat.
- The same procedure is replicated on the patient's left. Heaney retractor placement is then at the 2 and 8 o'clock position.

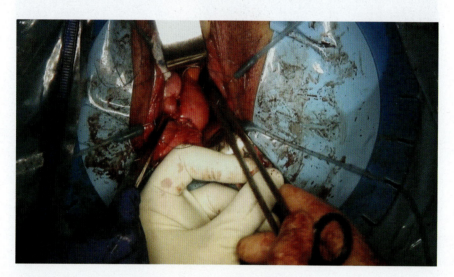

Tech Figure 2.4. Ensure lateral to medial placement of suture.

Ensuring Ureteral Integrity

- Cystoscopic evaluation for ureteral patency should be done prior to proceeding. The ureters reside within 1 cm laterally of the uterosacral ligaments. They are vulnerable to either injury or "kinking" with suture placement.
- Visualizing ureteral flow both without and with tension on the uterosacral ligaments is crucial. Obviation of this step or failure to identify ureteral obstruction prior to leaving the operating room can have a calamitous outcome for the patient (and physician).
- Intraoperatively if poor or absent ureteral flow is observed, simple removal of the suture is mandated. Identifying which of the two sutures requires some patience; however the offending suture once recognized can be removed and replaced in a more medial position. Once done cystoscopy should again be completed to confirm restoration of ureteral efflux.

Attaching the Vaginal Cuff to the Uterosacral Ligament

- Prior to affixing suture to the cuff, the anterior vaginal repair should be performed. Either traditional midline colporrhaphy or paravaginal repair can be done. Once completed, the associated anterior vaginal incision should be closed ⅔ of the way back to the original cuff incision. This will make final vaginal closure easier, as once the cuff is tied down, the vaginal incision will be in a more challenging elevated and inaccessible location.
- The technique of cuff affixation to the uterosacral ligament sutures, if done methodically, can be done with facility. All four uterosacral sutures should be in place prior to tying them down.
- Note each ligament has two sutures, one cephalad and one caudad.
- Starting on patient's right side, attach the lateral aspect, (9:00) of the cuff to the more cephalad suture (curved hemostat). This will allow maximal elevation of the vaginal cuff at the lateral margins (**Tech Fig. 2.5**).
- The suture should incorporate a portion of peritoneum and vaginal wall while avoiding coming through epithelium. A 0.5-cm margin from the cuff edge should be maintained to ensure the knot remains above the vaginal closure.
- The caudal suture (straight hemostat) can then be secured to the 10:00 position.
- A free needle can be then used for the non-needled suture and affixed to the 8:00 position.
- The same is completed on the contralateral side and the sutures tied down. This should elevate the cuff to its natural position.
- Completion of vaginal incision and cuff is performed.

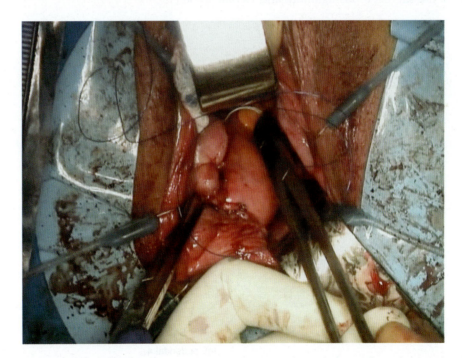

Tech Figure 2.5. Placement of right uterosacral ligament suture through the ipsilateral vaginal cuff.

Sacrospinous Ligament Vault Suspension

- This is one of the most utilized and studied techniques for fixation of the vaginal vault. Like a uterosacral ligament suspension, it can be done at the time of or remotely after hysterectomy for the treatment of apical prolapse. It is an extraperitoneal approach.

Incision and Exposure

- The incision is made on the posterior vagina and can include a wedge of perineal skin if a concomitant perineoplasty is to be performed.
- Dissection of the posterior vaginal epithelium is carried in cephalad direction to the vaginal apex and laterally to the rectal pillars. The rectum and its overlying endopelvic fascia are exposed.
- The ischial spine and associated sacrospinous ligaments are palpated. Using a combination of sharp and blunt dissection the rectal pillars are perforated. Dissection is carried down using manual palpation of the ligament. This leads to separation of the overlying thin, flat coccygeus muscle and the sacrospinous ligament can then be exposed.
- There are important neurovascular structures to avoid during dissection and suture placement. Most notably the pudendal artery, vein, and nerve course below the lateral aspect of the sacrospinous ligament and ischial spine (Tech Fig. 2.6).

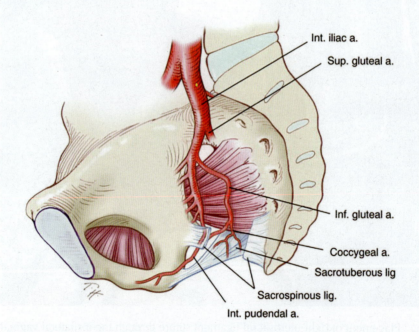

Tech Figure 2.6. Sacrospinous ligament vascular anatomy. Lateral view of pelvis and sacrospinous ligament and associated vascular anatomy. (Redrawn from Thompson JR, Gibbs JS, Genadry R, Burrows L, Lambrou N, Buller JL. Anatomy of pelvic arteries adjacent to the sacrospinous ligament: importance of the coccygeal branch of the inferior gluteal artery. *Obstet Gynecol*. 1999;94:973–977, with permission.)

Suture Placement

- There are several methods for suture affixation of the ligament with a number of instruments described over the decades that have been used to perforate the thick ligament since this technique was first described. Among them is included suture passage with a Deschamps or a Miya Hook with suture retrieval using a nerve hook (**Tech Fig. 2.7**). Contemporary options also include a Capio suture capturing device (Boston Scientific, Marlborough, MA), which allows one to both "push" and "catch" the suture requiring less exposure and dissection.
- Monofilament, permanent or delayed absorbable suture may be used.
- Specific placement of suture during this procedure is vital to avoid vascular or neural complications. Remaining at least 1.5 cm medial or one fingerbreadth to the tip of ischial spine should avoid pudendal nerve injury. One or two sutures may be used.
- Placement of suture in the body of ligament avoiding proximal placement avoids risk of injuring sacral nerve roots.
- The procedure is typically done unilaterally, but has been described with bilateral fixation though this in many cases may lead to suture bridge or undue tension on the cuff.

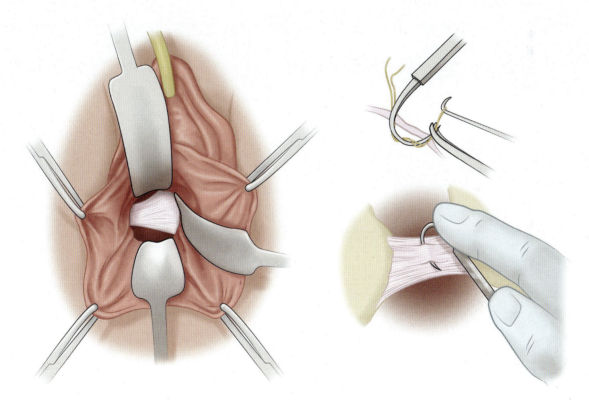

Tech Figure 2.7. Placement of suture through sacrospinous ligament using Miya Hook. (Adapted from Baggish MS, Karram MM. *Atlas of Pelvic Anatomy and Gynecologic Surgery*. New York: Saunders; 2001.)

Attaching the Vaginal Cuff

- The suture should incorporate full thickness vaginal wall while avoiding coming through epithelium. The sacrospinous ligament (SSL) suture should be attached to the associated apex of the vagina. The cuff is then tied down.

Uterine Sparing Technique for Apical Prolapse

- Many women would like the option of avoiding a hysterectomy in the management of their prolapse. Reasons forwarded to retain the uterus include not family complete, concern about impact on hormone function, wish to avoid perceived elevated risks of extirpation, concerns of adverse sexual function, desire to maintain cyclic menses, and loss of feminine identity. It is important to explore the reasons and discuss, particularly in women who perceive associated ovarian removal with the term "hysterectomy."

Uterosacral Ligament Hysteropexy

- The case is initiated in a fashion similar to hysterectomy with the exception that the cervicovaginal incision is limited to the posterior "hemisphere" of the vaginal fornix.
- Begin by infiltration of a mixture of 0.25% bupivacaine with 1:200,000 units epinephrine along the posterior vaginal epithelium at the level of the cervicovaginal junction from 3:00 to 9:00.
- An incision is carried through the epithelium, the epithelium advanced and the posterior cul-de-sac entered.
- The uterosacral ligaments are isolated and clamped. Then transected and suture ligated bilaterally.
- Next the bowels are packed away in a cephalad direction and then using a Heaney retractor, anterior retraction is implemented to retract the uterus and anterior vagina. The challenge is to create a large enough window to visualize suture placement.
- The posterior vaginal cuff is ipsilaterally grasped with Allis clamps and placed on traction.

Suture Placement

- The procedure is then carried out in a similar fashion as a traditional uterosacral ligament vault suspension.
- The middle finger of the surgeon's nondominant hand is placed in the rectum and with upward palpation toward the peritoneum the uterosacral ligament can be then identified. This should possess the tactile sensation of a thick guitar string and will be readily discernible even in the most lax of prolapse.
- A 2.0 monofilament, permanent or delayed absorbable suture, such as polypropylene or polydioxanone sulfate, is placed lateral to medial through the ligament. The first suture should be placed at the level of the ischial spine.
- A second suture of the same can then be placed 1 cm more cephalad than the previous. Both sutures are tagged and secured to the retractor frame with the needles still intact until time for fixation to the uterus/cervix.

Attaching Suture to Uterus/Cervix

- To adequately provide support the uterine cervix has avascular dense collagenous base to utilize.
- Place the more cephalad suture near posterior cervix midline and the caudal suture laterally on the cervix.
- When sutures are tied down both elevation and posterior displacement will occur.
- Avoiding tension and suture bridging are essential.
- Closure of vaginal cuff is done with a 2.0 absorbable suture.

PEARLS AND PITFALLS

UTEROSACRAL LIGAMENT VAGINAL VAULT SUSPENSION

- ○ Rectal examination with middle finger of nondominant hand with simultaneous posterior vaginal cuff traction is essential to adequately and reliably identify the uterosacral ligament (USL).
- ○ Cystoscopic evaluation both without and with traction to confirm ureteral function and patency is essential.
- ✗ Avoid using permanent braided suture to avoid exposure of suture through the vaginal skin and granulation tissue formation.

SACROSPINOUS LIGAMENT VAGINAL VAULT SUSPENSION

- ○ Precise placement of suture through the SSL at least 1.5 cm medial from the tip of ischial spine is important in avoiding nerve injury.
- ○ Attention to exposing the SSL with careful dissection will improve suture placement.

POSTOPERATIVE CARE

- As this is done in minimal invasive fashion, single night observation is recommended. Hysteropexy can be done as outpatient.
- Routine management with overnight bladder drainage and vaginal packing are suggested.
- Though there are limited data on activity restriction after vaginal reparative surgery, limiting chronic repetitive straining and heavy lifting is reasonable for 4 to 6 weeks.
- Pelvic rest for vaginal incision healing is also encouraged for a minimum of 6 weeks.
- Prevention of constipation to avoid straining during bowel movements is beneficial to healing.

OUTCOMES

Long-term outcomes of up to 5 years have been reported for uterosacral ligament suspension, with objective recurrent prolapse rates of 15.3% and subjective failure rates of 2.8%. In a review of 11 large-scale trials, sacrospinous ligament fixation success rates vary between 67% and 98%.

COMPLICATIONS

- Ureteral kinking is noted in up to 9% of uterosacral ligament suspension during cystoscopic evaluation intraoperatively. Identifying the offending suture at the time of surgery is essential.
- Neuropathy of pudendal nerve or sacral nerve roots can occur. Posterior gluteal, rectal, or thigh pain can all result from nerve entrapment or impingement. Most pain is self-limited and can be managed with nonsteroidal anti-inflammatory medications. However, if patients immediately complain of severe nerve pain in this pudendal or sciatic distribution then consideration of suture release should be entertained and pursued.

KEY REFERENCES

1. Barber MD, Visco AG, Weidner AC, Amundsen CL, Bump RC. Bilateral uterosacral ligament vaginal vault suspension with site-specific endopelvic fascia defect repair for treatment of pelvic organ prolapse. *Am J Obstet Gynecol*. 2000;183(6):1402–1410.
2. Gutman R, Maher C. Uterine-preserving POP surgery. *Int Urogynecol J*. 2013;24(11):1803–1813.
3. Karram M, Goldwasser S, Kleeman S, Steele A, Vassallo B, Walsh P. High uterosacral vaginal vault suspension with fascial reconstruction for vaginal repair of enterocele and vaginal vault prolapse. *Am J Obstet Gynecol*. 2001;185(6):1339–1342; discussion 1342–1343.
4. Leone Roberti Maggiore U, Alessandri F, Remorgida V, Venturini PL, Ferrero S. Vaginal sacrospinous colpopexy using the Capio suture-capturing device versus traditional technique: feasibility and outcome. *Arch Gynecol Obstet*. 2013;287(2):267–274.
5. Maher C, Baessler K, Glazener CM, Adams EJ, Hagen S. Surgical management of pelvic organ prolapse in women. *Cochrane Database Syst Rev* 2004; 18(4): CD004014.
6. Maher CF, Cary MP, Slack MC, Murray CJ, Milligan M, Schluter P. Uterine preservation or hysterectomy at sacrospinous colpopexy for uterovaginal prolapse. *Int Urogynecol J Pelvic Floor Dysfunct*. 2001;12: 381–385.
7. Morley GW, DeLancey JO. Sacrospinous ligament fixation for eversion of the vagina. *Am J Obstet Gynecol*. 1988;158(4):872–881.

Chapter 3
Posterior Vaginal Wall Repair
Erin M. Mellano, Lisa Rogo-Gupta

GENERAL PRINCIPLES
IMAGING AND OTHER DIAGNOSTICS
PREOPERATIVE PLANNING
SURGICAL MANAGEMENT
PROCEDURES AND TECHNIQUES
    Vaginal Approach
    Traditional Colporrhaphy
    Laparoscopic Approach for Posterior Vaginal Wall Prolapse
PEARLS AND PITFALLS
POSTOPERATIVE CARE
OUTCOMES
COMPLICATIONS

Posterior Vaginal Wall Repair

Erin M. Mellano, Lisa Rogo-Gupta

GENERAL PRINCIPLES

Definition

- Posterior Vaginal Wall (PVW) defect results from a weakness in the support of the posterior vaginal wall. The integrity of the posterior vagina is reliant on endopelvic fascia between the rectum and vagina, sometimes referred to as the rectovaginal septum. The rectovaginal septum consists of connective tissue composed of the lamina propria of the vagina, adventitial tissue and fibromuscular layers of both the vagina and rectum.
  - Rectocele is a common term used to describe PVW defects and is the prolapse of the rectum toward the anterior rectal and posterior vaginal wall into the lumen of the vagina (Fig. 2a) [17].
- PVW defects can be composed of different structures herniating into the vagina.
  - Rectocele (rectum presses into the vagina) (Fig. 3.1)
  - Enterocele (small bowel slides down between the vagina and rectum, resulting in a protrusion into the vagina) (Fig. 3.2)
- Posterior vaginal wall defects can be seen as isolated defects, or in combination with prolapse of the anterior vaginal wall or the apex (Fig. 3.3).
- Risk factors for posterior vaginal wall prolapse are similar to other types of prolapse and include:
  - Pregnancy
    - Vaginal child birth
    - Operative vaginal delivery
    - Prolonged second stage of labor
    - Large infant birth weight
  - Pelvic surgery/trauma
  - Conditions resulting in chronic elevated intra-abdominal pressure
    - Constipation
    - Chronic obstructive pulmonary disease
    - Elevated body mass index
  - Menopause
  - Genetics
- Symptoms of posterior vaginal wall prolapse include:
  - Sensation of bulge in the vagina
  - Pressure in pelvic area
  - Need to apply maneuver to defecate including:
    - Splinting to defecate on perineum or buttocks
    - Intravaginal digitation
    - Rectal digitation

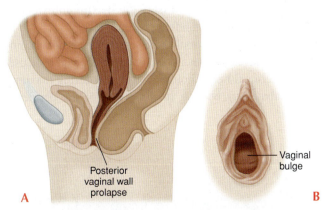

Figure 3.1. **A:** Sagittal view of a posterior vaginal wall defect, illustrating the rectum pushing into the vagina. **B:** Vaginal view of a posterior vaginal wall bulge. (Adapted from Knight L. *Medical Terminology: An Illustrated Guide Canadian Edition*. 2nd ed. Philadelphia, PA: Wolters Kluwer; 2013; Bickley LS, Szilagyi P. *Bates' Guide to Physical Examination and History Taking*. 8th ed. Philadelphia, PA: Lippincott Williams & Wilkins; 2003.)

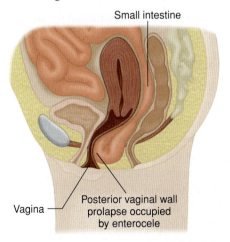

Figure 3.2. An enterocele occurs when the small intestine herniates between the rectum and the posterior vaginal wall. (Adapted from Berek JS. *Berek & Novak's Gynecology*. 15th ed. Philadelphia, PA: Lippincott Williams & Wilkins; 2012.)

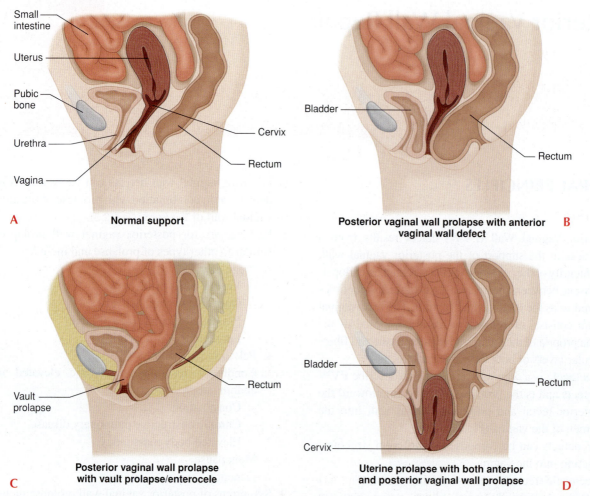

Figure 3.3. A, B, C, D: Posterior vaginal wall prolapse can be in isolation or in combination with other pelvic floor defects. This figure illustrates multicompartment prolapse. **A:** Normal pelvic floor support. **B:** Rectocele and cystocele. **C:** Enterocele. **D:** Uterine prolapse with cystocele and rectocele. (Adapted from Hatfield NT. *Introductory Maternity and Pediatric Nursing.* 3rd ed. Philadelphia, PA: Wolters Kluwer; 2013.)

- Defecatory dysfunction including:
  - Constipation
  - Sensation of outlet obstruction or "stool pocketing"
  - Fecal incontinence

Physical Examination

- Patient history and general pelvic examination: Please see Exam Table (Table 1.1).
- A focused neurologic exam should be performed to assess for any nerve deficits that may contribute to the posterior vaginal wall defect.
  - This exam should include:
    - The evaluation of sensation of sacral nerve roots 2–4 of bilateral lower extremities (Fig. 3.4)
    - Bulbocavernosus reflex
    - Anal wink
    - Pelvic floor strength assessment
- Pelvic organ prolapse quantification (POP-Q): Please see description of POP-Q (Chapter 1); it can be performed in the supine position.
- It can be helpful to assess the maximum extent of prolapse in the standing position.
- All compartments should be assessed, as it is not uncommon to have more than one compartment with prolapse.
- The perineal body should be assessed during maximal Valsalva. Any bulging or distension of the perineum

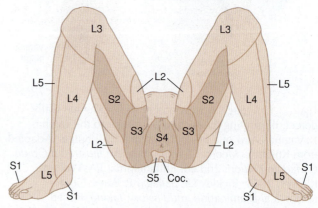

Figure 3.4. Dermatome distribution of the lower extremities and perineum.

should be noted. Concomitant rectal examination can reveal ventral distension of the anterior rectal wall pushing out toward the perineum or into the vagina.
- Rectovaginal exam should always be performed. This exam will help discern the area and size of the posterior vaginal defect and will help assess integrity of the anal sphincter. It will also allow for palpation of an enterocele sliding between vagina and rectum.
- If not easily assessed in the supine position, this exam can be repeated in the upright position.

Differential Diagnosis
- Vaginal vault prolapse
- Anterior vaginal wall prolapse
- Vaginal wall or vulvar cyst
- Functional bowel disorders

Nonoperative Management
- Expectant management is always an option for patients with minimal symptoms or for those who decline treatment.
- Bowel symptom management can be very helpful for women with defecatory dysfunction. It is not uncommon for the symptoms to have a functional component, and their symptoms may not correlate with the degree of prolapse.
  - For patients with chronic constipation, it is imperative to address this with dietary and medication modifications prior to any interventions, such as increased fiber, laxatives, and fluids.
- For patients with fecal incontinence, this also should be addressed.
  - Dietary bulking agents may help prevent the loss of loose stool
  - Antimotility agents, such as loperamide
  - Physical therapy, biofeedback, and/or electrical stimulation[1]
  - Sacral nerve root stimulation[2]
  - There is limited data to support the use of percutaneous tibial nerve root stimulation, and it is currently being investigated as a reasonable alternative to sacral nerve root stimulation.[3]
- Pelvic floor muscle exercises with or without physical therapy and biofeedback can be very helpful for improving bowel symptoms.
- Pessaries are the mainstay of nonoperative prolapse management. There are two classifications of pessaries: support devices and space filling. There is no consensus as to which pessary is superior for posterior vaginal wall prolapse. For prolapse in general, a ring with support style is most common for stage II/III prolapse; while for stage IV prolapse, use of a Gellhorn pessary may have improved success (Fig. 3.5).

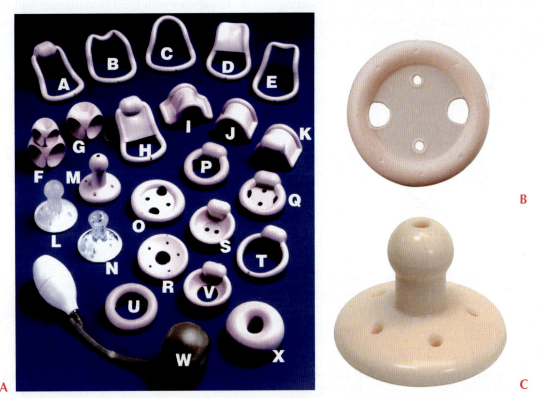

Figure 3.5. Pessaries come in many different shapes and styles. **A:** Depicts the wide variety of pessaries. (From Curtis M, Linares ST, Antoniewicz L. *Glass' Office Gynecology*. 7th ed. Philadelphia, PA: Wolters Kluwer; 2014.) **B:** Ring with support type pessary is the most frequently used pessary. (© 2017 CooperSurgical Inc. All rights reserved.) **C:** Gellhorn style pessary may be best for stage IV prolapse. (© 2017 CooperSurgical Inc. All rights reserved.)

- Gehrung or "saddle" pessaries can be used specifically for posterior vaginal support.
  - Unfortunately large posterior vaginal wall prolapse is associated with failure of initial pessary fitting.[4]

IMAGING AND OTHER DIAGNOSTICS

- When the clinical exam does not correlate with symptoms, diagnostic imaging can be helpful.

Defecogram

- A defecogram is a xeroradiographic study in which defecation can be observed real time with fluoroscopy. In this procedure, barium paste is instilled into the rectum and the patient is asked to defecate on a commode chair while serial images are obtained with fluoroscopy (Video 3.1).
- This imaging technique is ideal for evaluating efficiency of elimination and for clinically significant stool pocketing within a posterior vaginal defect.
- Defecograms describe:
  - The anorectal angle
  - Ability to completely evacuate rectal contents
  - Posterior vaginal defects
  - Perineal descent
  - Anal canal width and length
- This modality allows patients to defecate in a sitting position, which may simulate clinical symptoms more accurately.

Magnetic Resonance Defecography (Video 3.2)

- This technique allows for evaluation of the entire pelvic floor and viscera during Valsalva maneuver. It is useful for evaluation of pelvic floor descent and multicompartment prolapse. It is also useful for identification of an enterocele if clinical exam is not definitive.
- Typically this technique is done in the supine position, which does have limitations in replicating defecation, as some patients find it difficult to defecate in this position.
- Open magnetic resonance (MR) techniques allow for evaluation in a sitting position, circumventing this limitation.

Colon Transit Studies

- For patients with constipation, colon transit studies with sitz markers may be helpful to delineate slow transit and decreased bowel motility (Fig. 3.6).
- This information is especially informative for treatment planning and postoperative expectations.

Endoanal Ultrasound (Fig. 3.7)

- Evaluation of the anal sphincter complex with ultrasound allows for assessment of anal sphincter defects.
- In patients with fecal incontinence and posterior vaginal wall prolapse, identification of this defect is relevant for preoperative planning.

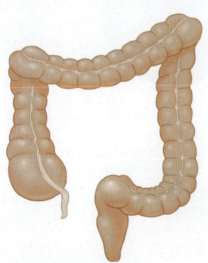 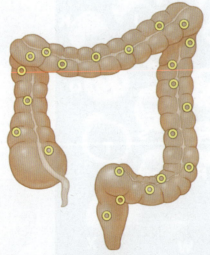 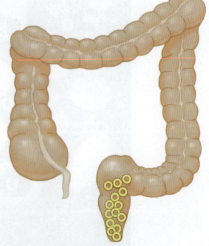

A If 5 or fewer markers remain, patient has grossly normal colonic transit.

B Most rings are scattered about the colon. Patient most likely has hypomotility or colonic inertia.

C Most rings are gathered in the rectosigmoid. Patient has functional outlet obstruction.

Figure 3.6. These images illustrate outcomes of a sitz marker study. **A:** Depicts normal transit time with all or the majority of the markers eliminated on day 5. **B:** Delayed colon transit time. **C:** Outlet obstruction with the majority of the sitz markers in the colon.

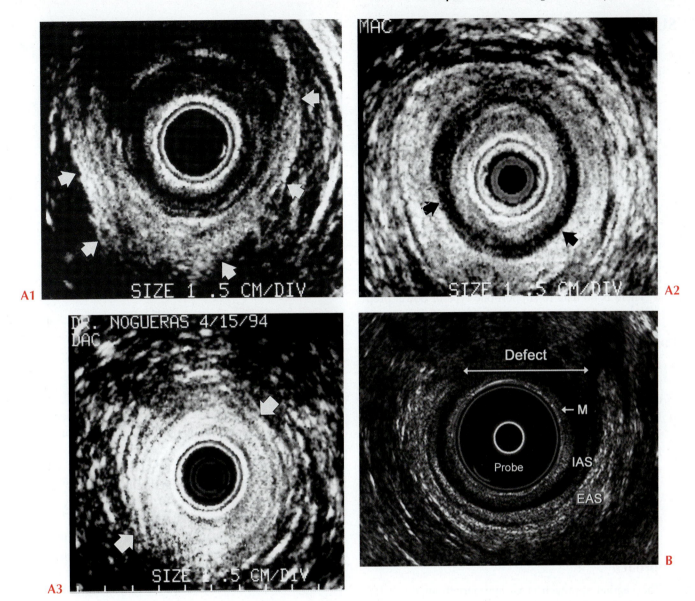

Figure 3.7. **A:** Image set A depicts a set of endoanal ultrasound images. 1 shows the upper anal canal with the puborectalis posteriorly (*arrows*). 2: Mid-anal canal with the hypoechoic internal anal sphincter (IAS) highlighted with *arrows* at maximum thickness. 3: Lower anal canal where the hypoechoic IAS has disappeared and is replaced by the hyperechoic external anal sphincter (EAS) (*arrows*). (Adapted from Corman C, Nicholls RJ, Fazio VW, Bergamaschi R. *Corman's Colon and Rectal Surgery*. 6th ed. Philadelphia, PA: Wolters Kluwer; 2012.) **B:** Image B depicts an anterior defect/tear in the EAS. The IAS is hypoechoic and intact. M = Subepithelial tissue. (From Rock JA, Jones HW. *Te Linde's Operative Gynecology*. 10th ed. Philadelphia, PA: Wolters Kluwer; 2008.)

PREOPERATIVE PLANNING

- Management of chronic constipation should be addressed prior to surgery, along with a discussion of postoperative constipation management strategies.
- For patients with a concomitant anal sphincter defect, discussion of plan for a concomitant repair can be considered.
- In patients with multicompartment prolapse, all compartments should ideally be addressed at the time of surgery.
- In patients with stress urinary incontinence, discussion should be had about options for concomitant repair.
- Rectovaginal exam can delineate area of defect in the fibromuscular tissue between the rectum and the vagina. In the instance of apical detachment of the fibromuscular tissue, apical suspension may aid in a site-specific repair.[5]
- Site-specific versus traditional posterior colporrhaphy.
    - Data does not support one technique over traditional approach.

SURGICAL MANAGEMENT

- Posterior vaginal wall defects are traditionally approached transvaginally. Alternatively, in patients with coexisting apical prolapse who elect to undergo a sacrocolpopexy, reinforcement of the posterior vaginal wall can be addressed with a sacrocolpoperineopexy.
- Colorectal surgeons may address these defects through a transanal approach; however there is level I evidence to support superiority in outcomes with transvaginal approach.
- For the purposes of this textbook, we will address only transvaginal and laparoscopic approaches.
- There is no data to support a preoperative bowel preparation; however, anecdotally surgeons request this of patients to eliminate stool from the rectum for purposes of intraoperative rectovaginal assessment.[6]
    - There is no data to support one type of bowel prep over another.

Positioning

- Regardless of transvaginal or laparoscopic approach, patients should be placed in the dorsal lithotomy position (**Fig. 3.8**).
- For vaginal procedures, arms may be left untucked for intravenous access.
- For laparoscopic procedures:
    - Patients should be placed in dorsal lithotomy position to allow adequate perineal access during the case.
    - The arms may be tucked to facilitate bedside access.
    - It may be beneficial to place an additional intravenous line to ensure adequate access during the case.

Approach

- The vaginal approach is an appropriate approach for most posterior vaginal wall defects.

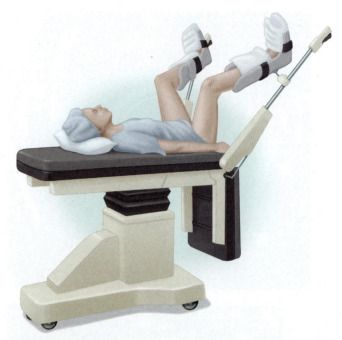

Figure 3.8. Lithotomy.

- Some surgeons prefer a transvaginal approach even if concomitant sacrocolpopexy is planned for apical prolapse.
- A sacrocolpoperineopexy can be performed laparoscopically and involves bringing the posterior vaginal mesh arm all the way down to the perineal body to support the posterior vaginal wall defect.
    - While data evaluating a posterior repair at the time of sacrocolpopexy found no difference in outcomes between the routes[7] there is some evidence to suggest that defecatory symptoms may be worsened after sacrocolpoperineopexy.[8]

Vaginal Approach

- This procedure may be done under regional or general anesthesia. The patient is placed in the dorsal lithotomy position. The vulva and vagina are prepped and draped.
- It is helpful to maintain access to the anus for rectal exam intraoperatively.
- A self-retaining vaginal retractor may be used to optimize visualization (**Tech Fig. 3.1**).
- If additional prolapse repair or incontinence procedures are planned, these are often performed prior to addressing the posterior compartment.
- A Foley catheter is placed in the urethra or the bladder is drained with an in and out catheterization.

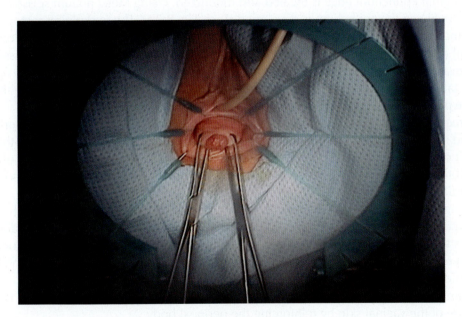

Tech Figure 3.1. Photo of a Lone Star self-retaining vaginal retractor.

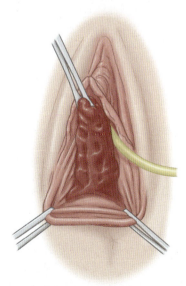

Tech Figure 3.2. This illustration depicts placement of Allis clamps for initiation of posterior colporrhaphy. This allows for tension to be placed for local infiltration of anesthetic with dilute epinephrine solution for hydrodissection.

Traditional Colporrhaphy

- Allis clamps are used to grasp the posterior fourchette at 5 and 7 o'clock. A third Allis clamp is placed midline at the apex of the prolapse.
- Local injection of bupivacaine or lidocaine with dilute epinephrine below the vaginal epithelium allows for hydrodissection and aids with hemostasis.
- If a concomitant perineorrhaphy is anticipated, a triangular wedge of epithelium and perineal skin is excised.
- If no perineorrhaphy is anticipated, a transverse incision at the junction of the vaginal epithelium and perineal body is performed (Tech Fig. 3.3A).
- The vaginal epithelium edge is created and mobilized. Using Metzenbaum scissors a plane between the epithelium is developed (Tech Fig. 3.3A). The underlying rectovaginal fibromuscular tissue is preserved. The vaginal incision is extended vertically to allow for lateral dissection of the vaginal epithelium off of the rectovaginal fibromuscular tissue until the levator muscles are reached (Tech Fig. 3.3B).
- A rectal exam should be done to ensure that the dissection was carried out above the level of the palpable defect.
- The rectovaginal fibromuscular tissue is plicated in the midline using delayed absorbable suture in an interrupted or figure-of-eight fashion (Tech Fig. 3.3C). This portion of the repair can be performed with a finger in the rectum to ensure adequate purchase of the fibromuscularis without traversing the rectum. Simultaneously this will allow for identification of areas of weakness.
- The vaginal epithelium may then be trimmed and closed in a running fashion with 2.0 delayed absorbable suture (Tech Fig 3.3D,E). There is no mandate to excise vaginal skin. When trimming the vaginal epithelium, care should be taken to prevent removal of too much epithelium, as this can narrow the vagina, put tension on the suture line, and cause chronic pain, particularly in postmenopausal females with atrophy.
- If a simultaneous perineorrhaphy was anticipated, this should be performed prior to closure of the vaginal skin by reinforcing the perineal body.

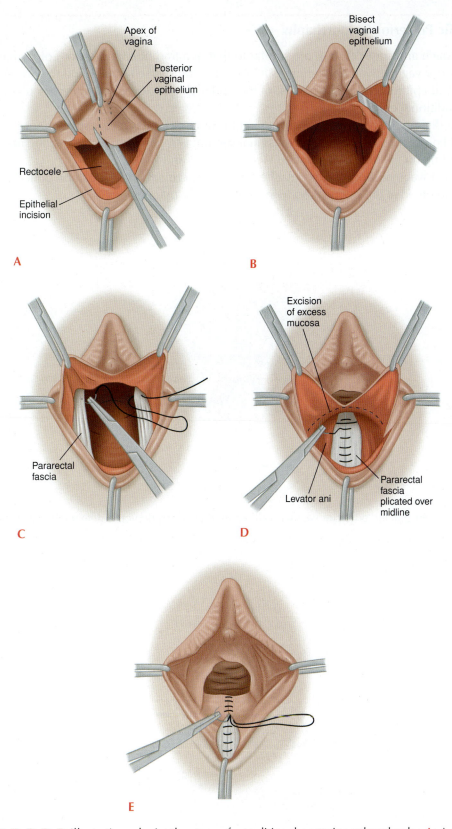

Tech Figure 3.3. A, B, C, D, E: Illustrations depict the steps of a traditional posterior colporrhaphy. **A:** A transverse incision is made in the posterior vaginal wall epithelium, just above the perineal body. The posterior vaginal wall epithelium is dissected off of the underlying fibromuscular tissue in the midline and a vertical incision is made. **B:** The posterior vaginal wall is dissected laterally off of the underlying fibromuscular tissue. **C:** The perirectal fascia/fibromuscular tissue is plicated across the midline, beginning above the site of the defect. **D:** If a concomitant perineorrhaphy is planned, the levator ani muscles and perineal body are reinforced. **E:** The vaginal epithelium and perineal skin are trimmed and closed in a running fashion.

Site-Specific Posterior Colporrhaphy

- The approach and surgical steps are similar to that of a traditional posterior colporrhaphy.
- The posterior vaginal wall epithelium is incised in a transverse manner and the posterior vaginal wall epithelium is dissected off of the underlying rectovaginal fibromuscular tissue as in a traditional colporrhaphy.
  - With a digit in the rectum the rectovaginal fibromuscular tissue is inspected for the area of weakness. The break in the rectovaginal septum is repaired in a site-specific manner depending on the area of disruption (**Tech Figs. 3.4** and **3.5**).
  - If the rectovaginal septum was detached from the perineal body, it can be pulled down and reinforced at the perineal body in a site-specific manner.

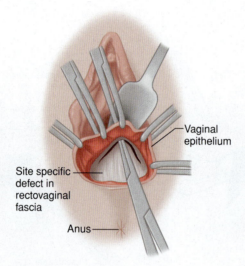

Tech Figure 3.4. Site-specific posterior vaginal wall repair. Illustration depicts a defect in the rectovaginal fascia.

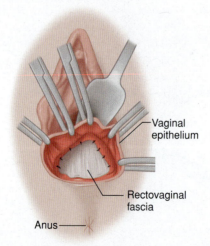

Tech Figure 3.5. Site-specific posterior vaginal wall defect repair. An approximation of the rectovaginal septum defect.

Apical Detachment (Video 3.3A,B,C ▶)

- Many posterior vaginal defects are the result of apical detachment of the rectovaginal septum. This can be easily identified with ventral distension during digital rectal examination **(Video 3.3 ▶)**.
- Reattachment of the rectovaginal septum to the apex with restore support. The sacrospinous ligaments are well positioned to serve as anchoring points for the rectovaginal septum when an apical defect is encountered.
- The posterior vaginal compartment dissection that was performed allows for easy access to the perirectal space. The ischial spine is palpated and the space is entered with blunt dissection.
- A suture capture device, such as a Capio can be used to place a permanent or delayed absorbable suture in the sacrospinous ligament.
- Sutures in the sacrospinous ligament should be placed one to two fingerbreadths medial of the ischial spine and care should be taken to not place the suture behind the ligament.
- Depending on the posterior vaginal wall defect, this suture can be placed on one side, or both sides, as indicated.
- This suture, or these sutures if bilateral, can then be used as an anchor for the apex of the rectovaginal septum.
  - The suture is affixed to the rectovaginal septum **(Video 3.3A ▶)**.
  - Once the rectovaginal septum is reinforced, the sacrospinous ligament sutures are tied down to correct the apical detachment of the rectovaginal septum **(Video 3.3B ▶)**.
  - Repeat exam demonstrates anatomic restoration and correction of the PVW defect **(Video 3.3C ▶)**.
  - The vaginal mucosa is trimmed as above, and the repair closed in a running fashion.

Graft Augmentation

- Transvaginal placement of synthetic polypropylene mesh in the posterior compartment does not improve the rate of a successful repair, and the risk of mesh erosion is unacceptably high.[9] At this time, it is not recommended to use transvaginally placed synthetic mesh in the posterior compartment.
- Augmentation with a biologic graft is reasonable when the fibromuscular tissue is obliterated and there is no tissue available to reinforce the defect.
- Data does not support improved outcomes with the use of biologic graft materials.[10]

Laparoscopic Approach for Posterior Vaginal Wall Prolapse (Video 3.4)

- The transabdominal route can be performed when there is a concomitant apical support defect. It can be approached with an open incision or with a laparoscopic procedure using a sacrocolpoperineopexy.
    - The patient should be placed in the dorsal lithotomy position.
    - The abdomen and the perineum should be prepped and a Foley catheter is placed into the bladder.
    - Laparoscopically this can be performed with or without robotic assistance and should be the surgeon's choice based on comfort level and patient characteristics.
- Intraperitoneal access is obtained and steps of a traditional sacrocolpopexy are initiated (Chapter 4: Apical Prolapse Repair: Abdominal Approach).
    - A vaginal manipulation device (such as an EEA sizer or Colpassist) is placed in the vagina to allow for dissection.
    - The peritoneum over the posterior vagina is incised and the rectovaginal space is dissected down to the level of the perineal body (**Video 3.4A**).
    - External pressure on the perineal body allows for laparoscopic identification (**Video 3.4B**).
    - The peritoneum of the posterior vaginal wall is opened and dissected all the way down to the perineal body.
    - The posterior mesh arm is affixed into the perineal body at the rectovaginal septum (**Video 3.4B**). The remainder of the posterior leaf of the mesh is affixed to the posterior vaginal wall using interrupted sutures.
- The remainder of the sacrocolpopexy is completed as described in Chapter 2: Vaginal Repair of Apical Prolapse.

PEARLS AND PITFALLS

CONSERVATIVE MANAGEMENT

- Use of a pessary is a reasonable conservative management approach.

DEFECATORY DYSFUNCTION

- Addressing bowel dysfunction prior to surgery is imperative. It may improve symptoms to a degree in which surgery is not necessary, and it will help manage postoperative expectations. It may be necessary to perform radiologic studies to best diagnose and treat the underlying defecatory dysfunction.

ROUTE OF SURGERY

- The preferred surgical route is via a transvaginal approach. If a simultaneous sacrocolpopexy is planned, it may be reasonable to perform a sacral colpoperineopexy. It would also be reasonable to perform the sacrocolpopexy as planned along with a transvaginal posterior colporrhaphy. The transanal route is not preferred.

TYPE OF POSTERIOR REPAIR

- Traditional posterior colporrhaphy and site-specific repairs have equal efficacy. The decision should be based on surgeon experience and preference. If an apical defect is present, this should be addressed to prevent recurrence. At this time, synthetic mesh grafts are not recommended.

POSTOPERATIVE CARE

- Bowel management is the most important element of postoperative care.

POSTOPERATIVE CARE

- Routine instructions for postoperative care are similar to that for other pelvic floor prolapse surgeries.
- **Foley catheter drainage**
    - There is no data to support postoperative use of a Foley catheter after an isolated posterior vaginal wall repair.
    - When patients undergo a posterior vaginal wall repair in addition to an incontinence procedure, anterior colporrhaphy, or vault suspension, we recommend leaving the Foley catheter in overnight and performing a void trial in the morning.
- **Antibiotic prophylaxis**
    - Antibiotic prophylaxis is not recommended after posterior colporrhaphy.
    - If mesh is utilized for a concomitant repair, antibiotic prophylaxis may be employed.
        - Antibiotic choice should cover gram-negative and gram-positive bacteria; however, no recommendation exists of type of antibiotic or of the dosing.
- **Bowel regimen:** *Recommended and required*
    - It is imperative that the patient avoids constipation in the postoperative period.
    - There is no data to support a particular bowel regimen.
    - If the patient is on a preoperative bowel regimen, this same regimen should be continued postoperatively.
    - To avoid straining, stool softeners should be utilized twice a day.
    - Additional laxatives can be added including polyethylene glycol daily, magnesium citrate, docusate sodium, or enemas.
- **Pelvic rest:** *Recommended and required*
    - Sexual intercourse or placement of any objects in the vagina must be avoided while the suture line heals. This typically takes 6 to 8 weeks.
- **Activity restrictions**
    - *Recommended:* There is no guideline on the particular amount of force that should be avoided postoperatively.
    - *Commonly done:* Avoiding heavy lifting of more than 10 to 25 lb is commonly recommended.

- **Follow-up visit for assessment**
  - *Commonly done*: There is no recommended interval for evaluation of patients after surgery. Typically patients are seen within at least 6 to 8 weeks. If a patient is having a complication, she should be seen promptly.
  - Long-term follow-up is dependent on surgeon preferences.

OUTCOMES

Midline Plication/Traditional Posterior Colporrhaphy

- Anatomic success rate varies between 76% and 96%.
- Postoperative dyspareunia ranges between 5% and 45%, and is thought to be highest with a levatorplasty.
- Up to 25% of women still need to digitally disimpact after repair.[11]
- Anatomic outcome does not always correlate with function.[12]

Site-Specific Posterior Vaginal Wall

- Success rates are reported at a similar rate to that of midline plication.
- In a retrospective comparison of site-specific to traditional plication, recurrence rates were significantly higher in the site-specific repair.[13]

Graft Augmented Repairs

- Graft augmented repairs (synthetic or biologic grafts) were compared in a prospective randomized controlled trial by Paraiso et al. He compared outcomes in women with site-specific, traditional colporrhaphy and graft augmented repairs. There was no significant difference in recurrence rates between the site-specific and traditional colporrhaphy; however, there was a significantly higher anatomic failure rate in the graft-augmented group at 1 year.[14]
- Increased morbidity was found with use of posterior compartment mesh with dyspareunia increasing in 63% of women, despite improved objective outcomes.[15]

Abdominal Repair With Sacrocolpoperineopexy

- Anatomic success ranges between 45% and 90%.[11]
- Symptomatic success rates vary from some studies reporting worsening function to others suggesting an improvement.[8,16–19]

Transanal Versus Transvaginal Approach

- Inferior objective results have been seen in the transanal group as compared to traditional colporrhaphy in a meta-analysis of several randomized controlled trials.[10]

COMPLICATIONS

Intraoperative Complications

- Bleeding
  - Use of a local anesthetic with dilute epinephrine or vasopressin helps to minimize bleeding during dissection.
  - Dissection into the perirectal space for a sacrospinous ligament fixation has the potential to result in bleeding that is difficult to control. This area should be packed for several minutes to attempt to control bleeding. If the vessel that is bleeding is identified, suture or clip ligation should be performed.
- Rectal injury
  - Inadvertent incision into the rectum is possible, especially if the patient has had prior repairs.
  - Bowel preparation does not minimize this risk.
  - Rectovaginal exam during dissection may help minimize the risk.
- Sutures placed into the rectum
  - Rectovaginal exam during suture placement will help minimize this risk.
  - At the end of the repair, a careful rectal exam should always be performed to ensure rectal patency and no sutures within the mucosa.

Early Postoperative Complications

- Vaginal bleeding
- Constipation and pain with defecation
  - Postoperative bowel regimen is essential to ensure no undo pressure is placed on the surgical repair.
  - Stool softeners should be given to all patients. In addition, laxatives and enemas may be used as needed.
  - Postoperative bowel regimen should be discussed prior to surgery.
- Infections
- Gluteal pain
  - Most specifically if a sacrospinous ligament suture is placed for apical detachment of the rectovaginal septum, gluteal pain may occur.
  - Mild buttock pain typically resolves in the postoperative period.
  - Severe buttock pain, accompanied by motor or sensory deficits should be addressed immediately, as this may be a reflection of suture entrapment of a branch of the sciatic nerve.
- Delayed complications
- Prolapse recurrence

- Defecatory dysfunction
  - De novo defecatory dysfunction has been reported after posterior colporrhaphy.
- Dyspareunia
  - More commonly occurs in women undergoing plication of the levators.

KEY REFERENCES

1. Vonthein R, Heimerl T, Schwandner T, Ziegler A. Electrical stimulation and biofeedback for the treatment of fecal incontinence: a systematic review. *Int J Colorectal Dis*. 2013;23(11):1567–1577.
2. Thaha MA, Abukar AA, Thin NN, Ramsanahie A, Knowles CH. Sacral nerve stimulation for faecal incontinence and constipation in adults. *Cochrane Database Syst Rev*. 2015;(8):CD004464. doi: 10.1002/14651858.CD004464.pub3
3. Edenfield AL, Amundsen CL, Wu JM, Levin PJ, Siddiqui NY. Posterior tibial nerve stimulation for the treatment of fecal incontinence: a systematic evidence review. *Obstet Gynecol Surv*. 2015;70(5):329–341.
4. Ramsay S, Tu le M, Tannenbaum C. Natural history of pessary use in women 65-74 versus 75 and older with pelvic organ prolapse: a 12-year study. *Int Urogynecol J*. 2016;27(8):1201–1207.
5. Glavind K, Christiansen AG. Site-specific colporrhaphy in posterior compartment pelvic organ prolapse. *Int Urogynecol J*. 2016;27(5):735–739.
6. Ballard AC, Parker-Autry CY, Markland AD, Varner RE, Huisingh C, Richter HE. Bowel preparation before vaginal prolapse surgery: a randomized controlled trial. *Obstet Gynecol*. 2014;123:232–238.
7. Grimes CL, Lukacz ES, Gantz MG, et al; NICHD Pelvic Floor Disorders Network. What happens to the posterior compartment and bowel symptoms after sacrocolpopexy? Evaluation of 5-year outcomes from E-CARE. *Female Pelvic Med Reconstr Surg*. 2014;20(5):261–266.
8. Ramanah R, Ballester M, Chereau E, Bui C, Rouzier R, Daraï E. Anorectal symptoms before and after laparoscopic sacrocolpoperineopexy for pelvic organ prolapse. *Int Urogynecol J*. 2012;23(6):779–783.
9. Schimpf MO, Abed H, Sanses T, et al; Society of Gynecologic Surgeons Systematic Review Group. Graft and mesh use in transvaginal prolapse repair: a systematic review. *Obstet Gynecol*. 2016;128(1):81–91.
10. Maher C, Feiner B, Baessler K, Schmid C. Surgical management of pelvic organ prolapse in women. *Cochrane Database Syst Rev*. 2013;(4):CD004014. doi: 10.1002/14651858.CD004014.pub5
11. Karam M, Maher C. Surgery for posterior vaginal wall prolapse. *Int Urogynecol J*. 2013;24(11):1835–1841.
12. Kahn MA, Stanton SL. Posterior colporrhaphy: its effects on bowel and sexual function. *Br J Obstet Gynecol*. 1997;104(1):82–86.
13. Abramov Y, Gandhi S, Goldberg RP, Botros SM, Kwon C, Sand PK. Site-specific rectocele repair compared with standard posterior colporrhaphy. *Obstet Gynecol*. 2005;105(2):314–318.
14. Paraiso MF, Barber MD, Muir TW, Walters MD. Rectocele repair: a randomized trial of three surgical techniques including graft augmentation. *Am J Obstet Gynecol*. 2006;195(6):1762–1771.
15. Milani R, Salvatore S, Soligo M, Pifarotti P, Meschia M, Cortese M. Functional and anatomical outcome of anterior and posterior vaginal prolapse repair with prolene mesh. *BJOG*. 2005;112(1):107–111.
16. Baessler K, Schuessler B. Abdominal sacrocolpopexy and anatomy and function of the posterior compartment. *Obstet Gynecol*. 2001;97(5 Pt 1):678–684.
17. Marinkovic SP, Stanton SL. Triple compartment prolapse: sacrocolpopexy with anterior and posterior mesh extensions. *BJOG*. 2003;110(3):323–326.
18. Fox SD, Stanton SL. Vault prolapse and rectocele: assessment of repair using sacrocolpopexy with mesh interposition. *BJOG*. 2000;107(11):1371–1375.
19. Thornton MJ, Lam A, King DW. Bowel, bladder and sexual function in women undergoing laparoscopic posterior compartment repair in the presence of apical or anterior compartment dysfunction. *Aust N Z J Obstet Gynaecol*. 2005;45(3):195–200.

Chapter 4
Apical Prolapse Repair: Abdominal Approach

Christopher M. Tarnay

GENERAL PRINCIPLES
PREOPERATIVE PLANNING
SURGICAL MANAGEMENT
PROCEDURES AND TECHNIQUES
    Abdominal Sacrocolpopexy
    Robotic-Assisted Laparoscopic Sacrocolpopexy
    Laparoscopic Uterosacral Ligament Suspension
    Hysteropexy
PEARLS AND PITFALLS
POSTOPERATIVE CARE
OUTCOMES
COMPLICATIONS

Apical Prolapse Repair: Abdominal Approach

Christopher M. Tarnay

GENERAL PRINCIPLES

Definition

Prolapse of the vaginal apex occurs when there are deficiencies in support of the upper portion of the vagina. The primary support structures involved are the uterosacral ligament and cardinal ligament complex. These structures have been described as level I support by DeLancey. Disruption or weakness of level I support during childbirth, trauma, or gynecologic surgery is considered to be the cause of apical prolapse (Fig. 4.1).

There are a number of terms that have been used to describe apical prolapse. When the uterus is in place: uterine prolapse, uterocervical prolapse; and in instances when vagina is completely everted: procidentia. When the uterus has been removed as in cases of hysterectomy, the terms: vault prolapse, cuff prolapse, enterocele, and apical prolapse are all described. Identification of apical defects is in general more difficult than other types of prolapse. This is because significant laxity of the apical vaginal support can exist but still visually remain above the vaginal opening. This is an important clinical consideration as the apex of the vagina is closely associated with the support of other vaginal compartments. Most relevantly the apex and the anterior wall are codependent and it is uncommon to have anterior vaginal laxity without concomitant apical descent. The surgical approach and correction of apical support remain a challenge for many surgeons.

In this chapter we will address apical prolapse repair using the abdominal route. This can include utilizing a laparotomy or a minimally invasive approach with laparoscopy. Using robotic assistance for laparoscopy is currently the most common technique to perform abdominal approach for vaginal apical prolapse.

Differential Diagnosis

- Anterior or posterior vaginal prolapse
- Vaginal wall cysts

Anatomic Considerations

Loss of apical support requires an understanding of the usual position of the cervicovaginal junction in normal support. The normal vaginal axis in a woman in the upright position is "banana" shaped. The distal third is near vertical with a sharp transition to almost horizontal for the upper vagina and rectum lying on and parallel to the levator plate (Fig. 4.2). Anatomic and imaging studies have placed the apex at approximately the level of ischial spines. Therefore attempts at restoration of normal anatomy should elevate a prolapse apex to near that location. Identifying surrogate structures to attach and resuspend the vaginal apex is requisite for anatomic restoration. Abdominally the uterosacral ligaments (USL) or the sacral promontory, specifically the anterior longitudinal ligament, are the two most reliable and most reproducibly identifiable structures used as an anchoring point for vaginal apex fixation (Fig. 4.3).

Removal of the prolapsed uterus via hysterectomy, combined with preventive procedures for future vault

Figure 4.1. Levels of support. In DeLancey classification the Level I represents the proximal support structures that include the uterosacral ligament and cardinal ligament complex. Procedures for apical support either must try to restore level I support by utilizing level I structures or find reliable surrogate such as the anterior longitudinal ligament of the sacrum. (Adapted from DeLancey JO. Anatomic aspects of vaginal eversion after hysterectomy. *Am J Obstet Gynecol.* 1992;166:1717–1724.)

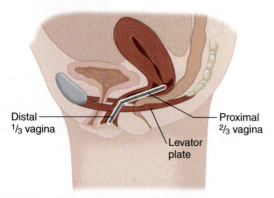

Figure 4.2. Sagittal view of the female pelvis. The vaginal axis in an upright woman demonstrates distal 1/3 in a near-vertical orientation with the upper 2/3 aligned in a horizontal position, laying on the levator plate.

prolapse, is considered the primary procedure in cases of uterine descent. With a vaginal approach, combined vaginal repair methods, such as anterior or posterior vaginal repairs, are easy to perform. If one chooses a vaginal procedure to correct uterine prolapse, one can choose to retain and suspend the prolapsed uterus rather than removing it, termed a hysteropexy.

Women have several reasons for wanting to preserve the uterus, such as retaining fertility and maintaining their personal identity. Other possible motivations may be the possibility that this kind of surgery might reduce operation time, blood loss, and postoperative recovery time.

Knowledge of the specific anatomy of the presacral space is critical. The risk of bleeding even catastrophic hemorrhage can occur if vascular structures are disrupted when the mesh fixation is not performed properly. Another rare but serious complication is spondylodiscitis that occurs when the vertebral disc is transgressed during suture placement. Spondylodiscitis refers to infection of the vertebral body and the intervertebral disc space.

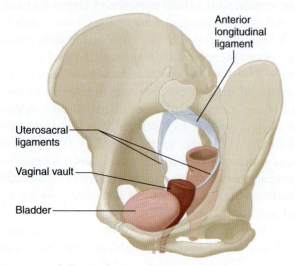

Figure 4.3. Abdominal view of options for anatomic fixation points of apical and vaginal vault prolapse.

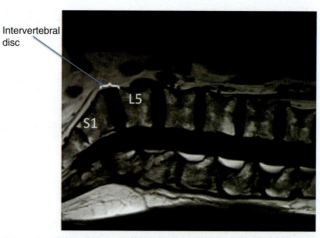

Figure 4.4. Intervertebral disc location during sacrocolpopexy.

In a study reviewing sacral anatomy on MRI in women undergoing sacrocolpopexy (SCP) the most prominent structure at the sacral promontory on MRI in women is often the intervertebral disc. The complexity of midline vasculature, as well as the proximity to major vessels and the right ureter, at this location, requires suture placement slightly below the promontory (**Fig. 4.4**).

Nonoperative Management

See Chapter 2: Apical Prolapse Repair: Vaginal Approach for nonoperative options.

PREOPERATIVE PLANNING

Proper patient selection is critical for optimal outcomes for prolapse correction. Apical prolapse should be demonstrated during clinical examination. Correlation with maximal extent of prolapse and the patient's own description of the prolapse severity should match. If there is a discrepancy, demonstrating maximal prolapse can be achieved by examining patient in the standing position. With patient standing and feet separated, maximal Valsalva and straining are performed and the prolapse can be elicited.

SURGICAL MANAGEMENT

The choice of operation for women with uterine prolapse should be tailored to her prolapse severity and be patient centered. The pelvic reconstructive surgeon should have all the requisite skills in one's "tool belt" to meet at minimum be able to offer a treatment plan to meet a patient's expectations. One needs to be mindful that ultimately conditions such as prolapse are almost never life threatening but *Quality of Life threatening*. The job of the pelvic reconstructive surgeon is to inform a patient of the options, provide available data and context, and arrive at a shared decision. Too often procedure selection depends on the inclination of the surgeon without balance for the preferences of the patient.

Chapter 4 Apical Prolapse Repair: Abdominal Approach

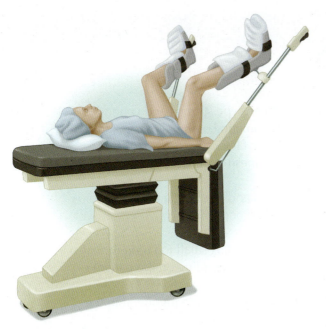

Figure 4.5. Lithotomy.

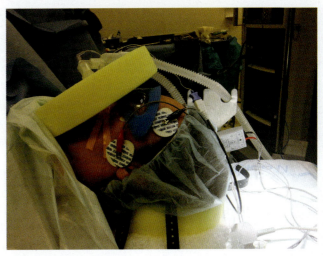

Figure 4.6. Face donut.

Uterosacral ligament vault suspension: performed by securing vaginal vault to the USL. This can be done during laparotomy after hysterectomy or via laparoscopy.

Sacrocolpopexy: performed by securing anterior and posterior vaginal walls via surgical mesh over the sacral promontory. Can be performed via abdominal or laparoscopic approach.

Positioning

- Abdominal apical support procedures via **laparotomy** can be performed with the patient positioned in low lithotomy (Fig. 4.5) with universal Allen-style stirrups. Perineal access is needed for vaginal manipulator placement to allow both mobility of the vagina as well as instrument-mediated vaginal distension to create of a backboard for suturing graft to vaginal walls.
- Abdominal apical support procedures via laparoscopy are also performed in dorsal low lithotomy with the same vaginal manipulator requirement as with abdominal approach but will often require steep Trendelenburg. Positioning is critical in robotic-assisted laparoscopy often requiring up to 30 degrees angle to allow for cephalad displacement of small and large bowel to facilitate view sacrum and pelvis.
- There are a variety of methods to secure a patient to prevent sliding toward the head during steep Trendelenburg utilized with robotic assistance. Use of foam "egg crate" pads or specially designed specific high-friction coefficiency pads are available. Safe-T-Secure (Chapel Hill, NC), Pink Pad (Xodus Medical) are two examples available.
- Nasogastric tube placement for gastric decompression may be helpful.
- Eye protection against corneal abrasion and face protection against camera port incidental contact should be used (Fig. 4.6).
- The arms should be tucked, with elbows padded and hands protected.
- The torso should be secured to the table.

Approach

The abdominal approach to uterine or vaginal vault prolapse was first described by Lane as a sacral colpopexy in 1962. This involved a laparotomy, a hysterectomy if uterus present, then fixation of the vaginal cuff to the anterior longitudinal ligament overlying the sacrum. Though initial description utilized the surface over S1 and S2, contemporary techniques utilize the sacral promontory, specifically the ligamentous covering—the anterior longitudinal ligament. This alteration was done to simplify dissection and most notably to avoid the rich venous plexus that exists in a more dorsal location. A graft would be used to attach to the anterior and posterior vaginal walls and the other end of the graft affixed to the anterior longitudinal ligament (Fig. 4.7).

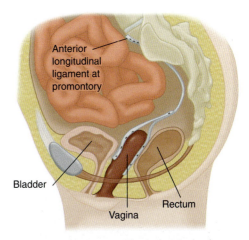

Figure 4.7. Sacrocolpopexy with graft attached to anterior vagina to trigone and posterior vagina to near perineum.

Abdominal Sacrocolpopexy

- With the patient in dorsal lithotomy position, universal Allen-type stirrups and venous thromboembolism prophylaxis in place in the form of pneumatic compression stockings plus heparin or low molecular weight heparin based on risk factors are provided. Prophylactic antibiotics should be used in all cases where mesh is utilized.
- A low transverse skin incision can be used.
- After peritoneal entry bowel is packed into upper abdomen and a self-retaining retractor is used. Anatomic survey with ureteral identification should be performed.
- A supracervical hysterectomy is completed.
- Use of a vaginal manipulator to distend fornices should be used. A small to medium malleable retractor, EEA sizer or vaginal stent can be inserted depending on the patient's vaginal capacity, cervix size, and sacral hollow space.
- Anteriorly the vesicouterine space is developed all the way down to the trigone. If in the proper space there should be minimal bleeding.
- Posteriorly the rectovaginal space is developed down to 4 to 5 cm below uterosacral ligament insertion. We find that skipping cervical peritoneum is often difficult to mobilize and can be skipped with incision beginning at more pliable fold caudally.
- At the level of the sacral promontory the iliac vessel bifurcation is identified. Importantly the relative position of the vena cava tends to be more caudal and slightly more to the right (**Tech Fig. 4.1**). Middle sacral vessels can also be visualized and desiccated or avoided.
- Dissection through the peritoneum over the sacral promontory is completed to expose the anterior longitudinal window. Usually a 1.5-cm window is sufficient.
- Two independent mesh pieces fashioned 4 cm × 10 cm or a "Y" mesh can be utilized.
- For open procedures, we begin anteriorly and place three to four pairs of sutures.
- Posteriorly the mesh is laid down and another three to four pairs of sutures are placed. The mesh should be flat and utilize the width of the vaginal wall.
- The mesh is laid into the hollow of the sacrum and secured to the anterior longitudinal ligament using two additional sutures.
- The mesh is retroperitonealized.

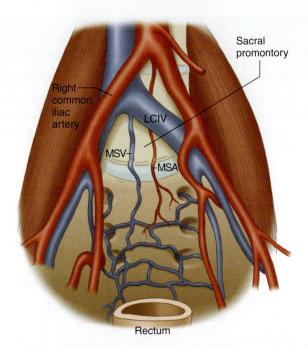

Tech Figure 4.1. Vascular anatomy of the presacral space. The bifurcation of iliac veins lay deep and caudal to the arteries. The left vein can be vulnerable to injury if not properly identified and avoided with sacral dissection during colpopexy. Also in the midline of the promontory is the middle sacral artery (MSA), middle sacral vein (MSV), and lateral sacral veins (LSV). (From Wieslander CK, Rahn DD, McIntire DD, et al. Vascular anatomy of the presacral space in unembalmed female cadavers. *Am J Obstet Gynecol.* 2006;195:1736–1741.)

Robotic-Assisted Laparoscopic Sacrocolpopexy

- Case initiation begins with placement of a Foley catheter, and if uterus present, a uterine manipulator with a cervix cup for forniceal delineation and occlusive cup over the stem to maintain pneumoperitoneum (Tech Fig. 4.2). For post-hysterectomy vault prolapse then vaginal manipulator is utilized (Tech Fig. 4.3).

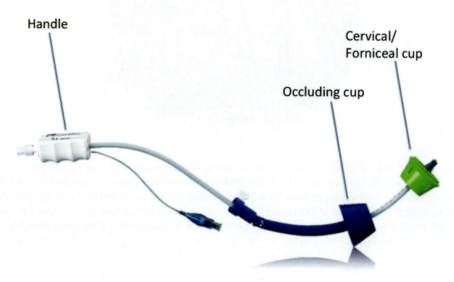

Tech Figure 4.2. Uterine manipulator. (Vcare. ConMed. Utica, NY.)

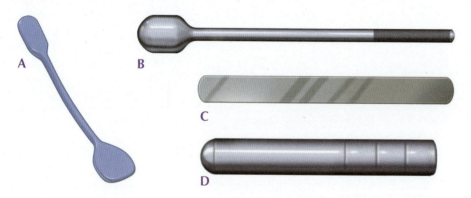

Tech Figure 4.3. Vaginal manipulators. A: Colpassist. (Boston Scientific, Marlborough, MA.) B: EEA sizer. (Courtesy of Victoria L. Handa. In: Jones HW, Rock JA. *Te Linde's Operative Gynecology*. 11th ed. Philadelphia, PA: Wolters Kluwer; 2015.) C: Malleable retractor. D: Stainless steel vaginal stent.

- Five total ports are utilized, although the procedure may also be completed with just four ports in some instances. For five-port technique a camera port is placed at the umbilicus. We prefer utilizing the cephalad border of the umbilicus to optimize sacral view. Three additional robotic ports are placed in either a "W" or "radial" configuration. Advantages of a "W" configuration placement (Tech Fig. 4.4) include easier separation of the ports and reduction of external arm collision. Using a "radial" configuration (Tech Fig. 4.5) will allow instruments more space to work within the pelvis and may be preferred for larger uterus. A fifth port is utilized as the assistant port and is usually located in right lower quadrant.

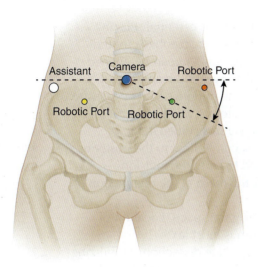 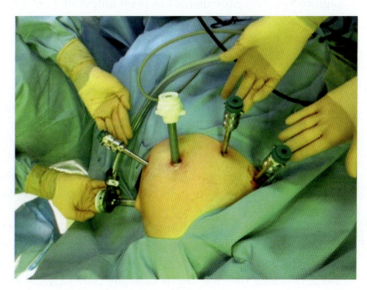

Tech Figure 4.4. Ports placed in a "W" configuration.

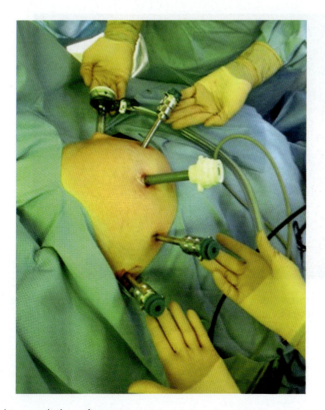

Tech Figure 4.5. Ports placed in a radial configuration.

- After peritoneal entry, for the hysterectomy and peritoneal dissection we employ a monopolar shear in primary port, bipolar forceps (or Maryland) in secondary port, and atraumatic grasper in tertiary port.
- A suggested first step is to orient the anatomy and identify feasibility of the procedure. Evaluating and accurately identifying the location and course of ureters (**Tech Fig. 4.6**), finding the sacral promontory, and ensuring the pelvis is free of adhesions are all critical steps prior to beginning case.
- If hysterectomy is required then completing uterine removal is done first. We advocate supracervical hysterectomy as a means to reduce mesh complications associated with vaginotomy. Once the uterus has been amputated off the cervix one may place corpus in upper abdomen for removal later.
- The sacral dissection is performed. Identification of the right ureter is essential. Placing proper location for incision can be facilitated by assistant using haptic feedback to find drop-off from promontory. Using monopolar energy the retroperitoneum can be opened and the underlying fat can be carefully desiccated down to the level of the anterior longitudinal ligament. There should be a white shiny surface. The middle sacral vessels are located typically just to the right of midline, though several anatomic variations have been described. Usually a 1.5-cm window is sufficient for fixation sutures (**Video 4.1**).
- The peritoneal incision can then be carried down along the sacral hollow to the posterior vaginal wall. Identifying the uterosacral ligament can be used to carry the incision caudally. The reflection of peritoneum will be used to cover the mesh at the completion of the case.
- Dissection can then be performed posteriorly over the rectovaginal space. Location of incision should be at the area where the overlying peritoneum is most lax.
- Strong traction and countertraction on the peritoneum will facilitate dissection. Mobilizing the peritoneum over the vagina caudally down toward the perineum and laterally to the uterosacral ligaments (USL) should be adequate for mesh placement (**Video 4.2**).

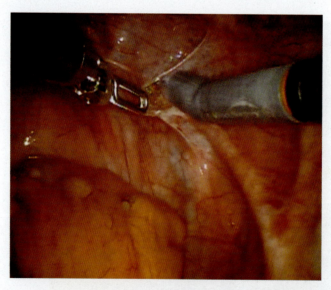

Tech Figure 4.6. Marking ureters on sidewall. Prior to initiating procedure, a marking incision over pelvic ureters is prudent for identification later in case.

- Adequate anterior dissection along the vesicovaginal space is necessary especially when coexistent anterior vaginal laxity exists. This should be carried down all the way to the level of the trigone. Careful identification of the plane between bladder and vagina is crucial to avoid inadvertent cystotomy. Conversely, one needs to avoid too thin a dissection on the vaginal wall to prevent mesh exposures and consequent complication.
- Use of a lightweight, knit, polypropylene type 1 mesh. This can be fashioned from a sheet into two "arms" or prefashioned into a "Y" (**Tech Fig. 4.7**). A common choice is polytetrafluoroethylene (ePTFE) Gore-Tex suture with a CV2 needle for all suturing.
- The mesh can now be affixed to the vagina. We prefer to start anteriorly. Initial placement is at the most distal site. A vaginal manipulator is used as a suturing backboard and to display the anterior segment. At least four pairs can be utilized (**Video 4.3**).
- Posterior mesh placement should be initiated near or as close to perineum to support posterior wall and reduce any existing prolapse of that segment. An additional four to five pairs of sutures should be placed.
- The sacral portion can be sufficiently secured with two sutures. To avoid going deep into cortical bone or injuring vessels avoid excess pressure allowing the suture to remain superficial and deflect along bony surface capturing ligament only.
- To avoid transgression of disc, suture placement just deep to promontory beginning close to S1 and performing in vertical orientation from a dorsal to ventral vector is preferred.
- Tensioning of the mesh for suspension can be accomplished in a variety of manners. There is no uniform technique though many have been described. Focus should be on avoiding undue tension as the purpose of the repair prolapse and preserving function. We prefer a neutral vagina. The vagina is placed on maximal cephalad displacement and then allowed to settle without pressure. It is this neutral position that is marked and suture affixed.
- The mesh is then retroperitonealized with an absorbable monofilament such as poliglecaprone 25 (Monocryl).
- If concomitant hysterectomy was performed it can be removed with contained tissue morcellation techniques.
- Cystoscopy is performed prior to completion to ensure bladder integrity and ureteral function.

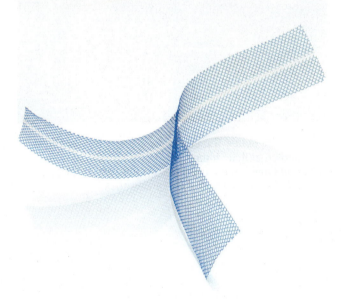

Tech Figure 4.7. Upsylon mesh.

Laparoscopic Uterosacral Ligament Suspension

- This technique is an excellent method for prophylactic vault fixation after hysterectomy for nonprolapse indications as well as a simple and secure method of addressing isolated apical prolapse. It can be easily performed with a cervix in place after supracervical hysterectomy or after total hysterectomy.
- Begin by identifying course and track of ureters. They will be running over the pelvic brim at the bifurcation of the internal iliac. The ureter then courses across the pelvic sidewall dorsal to the infundibulopelvic ligament and lateral to the uterosacral ligament (Tech Fig. 4.8).
- To facilitate identification of the USL one needs to place the posterior peritoneum on traction. This can be accomplished via upward displacement of the vaginal cuff ventrally toward anterior abdominal wall or by cephalad traction on the posterior peritoneum near the sacrum. Using a vaginal manipulator is helpful. This will accentuate the USL.
- In general the right USL is easier to visualize and access as sigmoid often overlies the left pelvic sidewall.
- Use of a monofilament permanent suture such as 2.0 polypropylene (Prolene) or delayed absorbable such as polydioxanone suture (PDS).

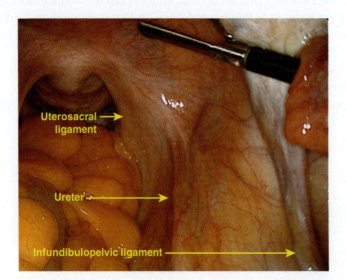

Tech Figure 4.8. Identification of the ureter. The ureter can usually be identified crossing the pelvic brim at the bifurcation of the internal iliac. It then courses across the pelvic sidewall dorsal to the infundibulopelvic ligament and lateral to the uterosacral ligament. (From Jones HW, Rock JA. *Te Linde's Operative Gynecology*. 11th ed. Philadelphia, PA: Wolters Kluwer; 2015.)

- Suspension can be initiated at the USL with a suture placed in lateral to medial vector. Ipsilateral placement at the level of cuff/cervix from posterior to anterior then return through from posterior to anterior to ensure adequate tissue purchase. The suture is then brought back down through ligament and can be tied (**Tech Fig. 4.9**).
- The same is performed on contralateral side.

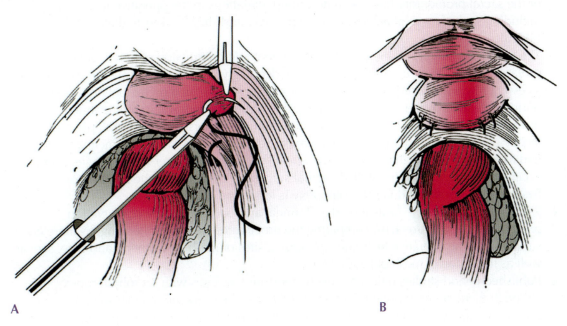

Tech Figure 4.9. Laparoscopic uterosacral ligament suspension. Two uterosacral ligament permanent sutures are placed through the deep portion of the ligament and to the ipsilateral vaginal cuff/cervix. **A:** Placement of right uterosacral ligament suspension suture to vaginal apex at the lateral margin. Care is taken to avoid the ureter laterally. **B:** Four total uterosacral ligament sutures have been tied, resuspending the vagina. (From Gibbs RS, Karlan BY, Haney AF, Nygaard IE. *Danforth's Obstetrics and Gynecology*. 10th ed. Philadelphia, PA: Wolters Kluwer; 2008.)

Hysteropexy

- Abdominally, procedures supporting the uterus/cervix to either the uterosacral ligament or the sacral promontory have been described. Variations in the operative technique, including sites of mesh attachment, and type, size, and shape of mesh, make comparison difficult.
- The role of the uterus, on the actual development and progression of pelvic organ prolapse has not been established. One may deem a typical menopausal sub–100 g organ as essentially a nonfactor given the existent pressures generated on the pelvic support during daily activities. The traditional inclusion of uterine removal in the treatment of vaginal prolapse is likely a consequence of limited understanding of prolapse and legacy procedures. Certainly for vaginal approaches uterine removal is a means to an end to adequately visualize and access pelvic structures. However vaginal hysteropexy is certainly plausible for the skilled vaginal surgeon. Persistence of the addition of hysterectomy for the abdominal colpopexy is less clear.
- Sacrohysteropexy is the best-studied abdominal approach of uterine conservation procedures. Tech Figure 4.10, comparing the procedures can be challenging, as there are variations in the operative technique, including sites of mesh attachment, and type, size as well as the shape of mesh utilized.
- Published cohort studies reflect relatively good success rates with sacrohysteropexy, although there are no randomized controlled trials. The outcome of laparoscopic sacrohysteropexy is limited but in a retrospective study by Pan et al. comparing laparoscopic hysteropexy to sacrocolpopexy after hysterectomy, objective cure rates were similar after 1 year.
- The abdominal uterine sparing technique we offer is robotic-assisted laparoscopic sacrohysteropexy. This procedure utilizes the same overarching principles as sacrocolpopexy. A "Y" mesh with two mesh arms are utilized with the added modification that the anterior piece is bisected and the two resultant arms perforate the broad ligament from behind and wrap anteriorly over the cervix and upper vagina **(Video 4.4)**.
- Laparoscopic uterosacral hysteropexy is performed in a similar fashion as the vault suspension with no additional dissection required.

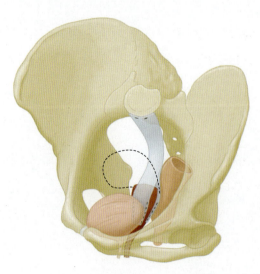

Tech Figure 4.10. Sacrohysteropexy. Apical support of the uterus and cervix using a graft to the anterior longitudinal ligament over sacral promontory. Can be performed via laparotomy or laparoscopic approach.

PEARLS AND PITFALLS

PATIENT POSITIONING

○ For steep Trendelenburg ensures patient perineum placed at bed break. Reduction of patient sliding can be facilitated with the use of secure and high-friction coefficient padding.

PORT POSITIONING FOR ROBOTIC ASSISTANCE

○ To avoid external instrument contact ensure ports separated by a minimum of 8 cm. To avoid incisional pain, keep lateral port location at least 3 to 4 cm from anterior superior iliac spine.

PRESACRAL SPACE

○ Severe hemorrhage can occur if disruption of presacral venous plexus over S1 or dissection carried too far cephalad into the iliac vein. Be mindful not to place suture just post to promontory and remain superficial through ligament only to avoid transgression of disc.

UTERINE PRESERVATION (HYSTEROPEXY)

○ Hysterectomy is not a mandate during apical repair. A discussion about the option of uterine preservation with a candid review of potential merits and limitations in outcomes data can be explored with patients.

COLPOPEXY MESH TENSIONING

○ Though no consensus exists for tensioning techniques, avoidance of an over tensioning and a taut vagina can avoid concern for sexual dysfunction postoperatively.

VAGINAL MANIPULATION

○ Regardless of technique, vaginal manipulators can assist in optimal vaginal positioning for apical fixation and colpodistension during suturing.

POSTOPERATIVE CARE

- After minimally invasive surgery most patient can be discharged within 24 hours even when hysterectomy performed.
- We maintain broad spectrum antibiotics for 24 hours when mesh graft is utilized.
- Bladder drainage can be discontinued within 24 hours. When concomitant mid-urethral sling is performed then assessment of adequate bladder empting is added with evaluation of post-void residual urine.
- Early ambulation, reintroduction of regular diet, and oral analgesics are all introduced soon after surgery.
- As with all prolapse correction surgery, activity is limited to avoid chronic repetitive straining during recuperation. Implementing constipation prevention strategies is important to preserve integrity of repair and allow healing.

OUTCOMES

- Robotic sacrocolpopexy
  - Follow-up duration for most studies ranged from 6 months to 3 years. The success rate, when defined as a lack of apical prolapse postoperatively, ranged from 78% to 100%, and when defined as a no-postoperative prolapse, from 58% to 100%.
  - In a long-term single institution review freedom from repeat prolapse surgery or surgery for mesh complication was 98% at 1 year, 95% at 3 years and 90% at 6 years. At last follow up, 80% of patients reported that they would or probably would recommend robotic sacrocolpopexy to a family member or friend.
  - Comparative trials evaluating laparoscopic sacrocolpopexy (LSC) versus robotic-assisted laparoscopic sacrocolpopexy (RALSC) note clinical outcomes of

prolapse surgery are similar but RALSC is less efficient in terms of cost and time.
- Laparoscopic uterosacral ligament repair of vault:
  - Rardin et al. reported a retrospective review of 22 women and found no significant differences in perioperative morbidity or anatomical or subjective outcomes when compared to vaginal uterosacral ligament suspension.
- Hysteropexy
  - Sacrohysteropexy
    - Open sacrohysteropexy is well described but has limited prospective data. Retrospective studies describe long-term success with no prolapse beyond hymen of 93% over 3 years. In two small prospective studies 95% of women had no prolapse after 24 months.
    - Laparoscopic sacrohysteropexy also has a paucity of data. Small studies demonstrate excellent results with <10% recurrence at 12 months.
    - In a study comparing laparoscopic or robotic sacrohysteropexy (RLSH) versus open sacrohysteropexy (OSH), the RLSH group had shorter operating time, less operative bleeding, and fewer postoperative symptoms. Overall satisfaction required reoperation due to postoperative complications did not differ between groups.
  - Laparoscopic Uterosacral Hysteropexy
    - Haj et al. reported anatomical cure, defined as no prolapse within a centimeter of the hymen was 85.4%. Clinical cure, defined as a composite outcome of no prolapse outside the hymen, C point above total vaginal length/2, no prolapse symptoms, and no need for further treatment, was 95.8%
    - In a systematic review that included a total of 770 patients in 17 studies, the subset of women undergoing laparoscopic suture uterosacral hysteropexy had a pooled success of 70.5%

COMPLICATIONS

- Complications of sacrocolpopexy procedures have been well documented which include mesh erosion, infection, severe hemorrhage, and pelvic pain. Uncommon complications such as spondylodiscitis and osteomyelitis have also been described.
- Ureteral complications.

SUGGESTED READINGS

Abernethy M, Vasquez E, Kenton K, Brubaker L, Mueller E. Where do we place the sacrocolpopexy stitch? A magnetic resonance imaging investigation. *Female Pelvic Med Reconstr Surg*. 2013;19:31–33.

Anger JT, Mueller ER, Tarnay C, et al. Robotic compared with laparoscopic sacrocolpopexy: a randomized controlled trial. *Obstet Gynecol*. 2014;123:5–12.

Barber MD, Maher C. Apical prolapse. *Int Urogynecol J*. 2013;24:1815–1833.

Bradley S, Gutman RE, Richter LA. Hysteropexy: an Option for the Repair of Pelvic Organ Prolapse. *Curr Urol Rep*. 2018;19(2):15. doi: 10.1007/s11934-018-0765-4. Review. PubMed PMID: 29476274.

Dietz V, Schraffordt Koops SE, van der Vaart CH. Vaginal surgery for uterine descent; which options do we have? A review of the literature. *Int Urogynecol J Pelvic Floor Dysfunct*. 2009;20:349–356.

Hagen S, Stark D. Conservative prevention and management of pelvic organ prolapse in women. *Cochrane Database Syst Rev*. 2011;(12):CD003882.

Haj Yahya R, Chill HH, Herzberg S, Asfour A, Lesser S, Shveiky D. Anatomical Outcome and Patient Satisfaction After Laparoscopic Uterosacral Ligament Hysteropexy for Anterior and Apical Prolapse. *Female Pelvic Med Reconstr Surg*. 2017;27. doi: 10.1097/SPV.0000000000000446. [Epub ahead of print] PubMed PMID: 28658003.

Linder BJ, Chow GK, Elliott DS. Long-term quality of life outcomes and retreatment rates after robotic sacrocolpopexy. *Int J Urol*. 2015;22(12):1155-1158. doi: 10.1111/iju.12900. Epub 2015 Aug 24. PubMed PMID: 26300382.

Nichols DH, Milley PS, Randall CL. Significance of restoration of normal vaginal depth and axis. *Obstet Gynecol*. 1970;36:251–256.

Nygaard IE, McCreery R, Brubaker L, et al; Pelvic Floor Disorders Network. Abdominal sacrocolpopexy: a comprehensive review. *Obstet Gynecol*. 2004;104(4):805–823.

Paek J, Lee M, Kim BW, Kwon Y. Robotic or laparoscopic sacrohysteropexy versus open sacrohysteropexy for uterus preservation in pelvic organ prolapse. *Int Urogynecol J*. 2016;27:593–599.

Pan K, Cao L, Ryan NA, Wang Y, Xu H. Laparoscopic sacral hysteropexy versus laparoscopic sacrocolpopexy with hysterectomy for pelvic organ prolapse. *Int Urogynecol J*. 2016;27:93–101.

Pan K, Zhang Y, Wang Y, Xu H. A systematic review and meta-analysis of conventional laparoscopic sacrocolpopexy versus robot-assisted laparoscopic sacrocolpopexy. *Int J Gynaecol Obstet*. 2016;132(3):284-291. doi: 10.1016/j.ijgo.2015.08.008. Epub 2015 Dec 9. Review. PubMed PMID: 26797199.

Ridgeway BM, Cadish L. Hysteropexy: evidence and insights. *Clin Obstet Gynecol*. 2017;60(2):312–323.

Rosenblatt PL, Chelmow D, Ferzandi TR. Laparoscopic sacrocervicopexy for the treatment of uterine prolapse: a retrospective case series re-port. *J Minim Invasive Gynecol*. 2008;15:268–272.

Wu JM, Matthews CA, Conover MM, Pate V, Jonsson Funk M. Lifetime risk of stress urinary incontinence or pelvic organ prolapse surgery. *Obstet Gynecol*. 2014;123:1201–1206.

Chapter 5
Urinary Incontinence Procedures

Lisa Rogo-Gupta, Christopher M. Tarnay

GENERAL PRINCIPLES
IMAGING AND OTHER DIAGNOSTICS
PREOPERATIVE PLANNING
SURGICAL MANAGEMENT
PROCEDURES AND TECHNIQUES
    Mid-Urethral Slings
    Pubovaginal Slings
    Transurethral Bulking
    Sacral Neuromodulation
    Sacral Neuromodulation: Special Considerations
PEARLS AND PITFALLS
POSTOPERATIVE CARE
OUTCOMES
COMPLICATIONS

Urinary Incontinence Procedures

Lisa Rogo-Gupta, Christopher M. Tarnay

GENERAL PRINCIPLES

Definition

- Urinary incontinence (UI) is involuntary loss of urine. The two most common types are stress (SUI), loss of urine with physical activity, sneezing, or coughing, and urgency (UUI), loss of urine associated with a sensation of urgency. Patients with features of both types are said to have mixed incontinence (MUI).
- There are two general types of injuries that result in symptomatic SUI.
    - Vaginal childbirth injury resulting in loss of urethral support. A physical examination finding of urethral hypermobility is typical of this diagnosis.
    - Urethral sphincter damage from lack of estrogen, radiation, aging, or surgery. Finding a fixed, open urethra at rest, or "lead-pipe urethra," is typical of this diagnosis.
- UUI may be associated with contractions or spasms of the bladder detrusor muscle. Patients feel an urgency to urinate that cannot be deferred for fear of leakage or discomfort. This sensation is distinct from the patient's normal sensation to urinate.
- Bladder storage symptoms may also be present in patients with UI, but not all patients with storage symptoms experience urine leakage. Storage symptoms include increased daytime frequency, nocturia, and urgency.
    - *Urinary frequency* is a bothersome increase in the number of urinations during the day compared to previous.
    - *Nocturia* is a bothersome increase in the number of urinations during the night compared to previous. Waking is for urination alone and not due to other causes such as sleep disturbances.
    - *Overactive bladder syndrome* is characterized by urinary urgency, typically with frequency and nocturia, with or without UUI, in the absence of urinary tract infection or other obvious pathology. UI may or may not be present.

Physical Examination

- General pelvic examination (see **Table 5.1**).
- Demonstration of SUI on examination involves visualization of involuntary urine loss with physical exertion. This can be performed with the patient in the supine or standing position.
- Urethral hypermobility can be demonstrated by placing a cotton swab (or urethral catheter) in the urethra and watching the patient cough or Valsalva. A change in angle of greater than 30 degrees is described as urethral hypermobility.
- Assess urogenital health by visualizing perineum, labial architecture, and appearance of urethral meatus. Erythema, inflammation, and especially vulvovaginal atrophy may adversely impact bladder function and control.
- Post-void residual (PVR) is the measurement of urine in the bladder following urination by transabdominal ultrasound or by catheterization. PVR assessment should be performed when considering surgical management of UI.
- Urinalysis or culture should be performed to rule out urinary tract infection in patients with UI considering surgical management, as infections are a common cause of UI.[1]

Differential Diagnosis

- Other causes of UI are easily remembered by the pneumonic **DIAPER**.
    - **D**elirium
    - **I**nfection (cystitis, urethritis, pyelonephritis)
    - **I**nflammation
    - **I**mpaction
        - Stool
        - Urine (urinary retention)
        - Vaginal foreign body
    - **A**trophic vaginitis or urethritis
    - **P**harmaceutical
        - α-Adrenergic agents
        - Diuretics
        - Narcotics and sedatives
        - Psychotropics
    - **E**xcessive urine production
        - Poorly controlled diabetes with glucosuria
        - Alcohol use
        - Edema (any etiology)
    - **R**estricted mobility

Table 5.1 Physical Examination for Patients Undergoing Urogynecologic Surgery

Organ System	Examination Findings		
General	Signs of systemic illness Peripheral edema		
Skin	Ecchymosis, ulcerations, rashes, changes in pigmentation		
Gynecologic	External female genitalia Glands (Skene, Bartholin) Urethral meatus Vaginal wall appearance (scarring, ulcers, lesions) Cervix and uterus (appearance, size, mobility, masses, tenderness) Adnexa (mobility, masses, tenderness) Rectum (anal tone, rectovaginal septum)		
Neurologic	Sensory evaluation (if indicated)		
Musculoskeletal	Mobility, ambulation, strength		
Additional	Post-void residual Urinalysis Bladder diary (or "voiding log")		
Pelvic organ prolapse	Anterior, apical, and posterior compartments Relax and strain positions		
Urethral hypermobility	Urethral mobility during Valsalva Hypermobility defined as ≥30 degrees		
Urinary incontinence	Involuntary leakage during Valsalva or with associated urge		
Pelvic floor evaluation	Tenderness, strength Perineal body and levator ani		
	0	Lack of muscle response	
	1	Flicker of nonsustained contraction	
	2	Presence of low-intensity, but sustained contraction	
	3	Moderate contraction, felt like an increase in intravaginal pressure, which compresses the fingers of the examiner with small cranial elevation of the vaginal wall	
	4	Satisfactory contraction, compressing the fingers of the examiner with elevation of the vaginal wall toward the pubic symphysis	
	5	Strong contraction, firm compression of the examiner's fingers with positive movement toward the pubic symphysis	
Fistula evaluation	Tampon test Imaging studies using intravenous or intrarectal contrast		

Adapted from Laycock J. Clinical evaluation of the pelvic floor. In: Schussler B, Laycock J, Norton P, Stanton SL, eds. *Pelvic Floor Re-education*. London, United Kingdom: Springer-Verlag; 1994:42–48.

Nonoperative Management

- Behavior and lifestyle modifications are considered first-line management for UI. These include weight loss, physical activity, fluid restriction, and timed voiding.
- Particular attention should be given to dietary intake of beverages or even foods that may contribute to bladder control difficulty. Triggers such as caffeinated beverages, carbonated beverages, alcohol, spicy foods, and citrus juices have all been associated with overactive bladder symptoms and even UI (see **Table 5.2**).

Table 5.2 Potential Dietary Bladder Triggers

- Citrus fruit juices (orange juice and grapefruit juice especially)
- Caffeine (coffee, including decaffeinated coffee)
- Carbonated beverages (coke, pepsi, and similar cola sodas)
- Tea (black and green tea)
- Alcoholic beverages
- Spicy foods, avoid cayenne and peppers
- Tomatoes (including the spicy sauces and tomato juice)
- Artificial sweeteners (aspartame, erythritol, saccharin, sucralose, xylitol)
- Cranberry juice (can worsen frequency because of the acidity)
- Vinegar (contained in many condiments)

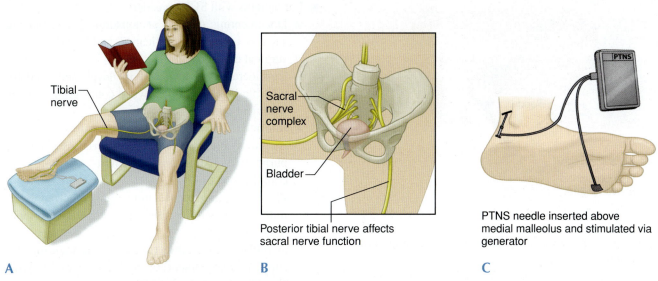

Figure 5.1. Posterior tibial nerve stimulation session. (Adapted from Graham SD, Keane TE. *Glenn's Urologic Surgery*. 8th ed. Philadelphia, PA: Wolters Kluwer; 2015.)

- Exacerbating factors should be controlled. These may include medications (type, timing, and dosage), sleep disturbances such as sleep apnea, mobility restrictions, and proximity to toilet facilities.
- Pelvic floor muscle exercises (PFME) have demonstrated effectiveness in the treatment of UI. PFME are an important first-line therapy for both mild to moderate SUI and UUI. Though women may have performed PFME in the past (commonly known as "Kegel" exercises), many are unable to assess proper performance or expected outcome. Physical therapy of the pelvic floor often coupled with biofeedback may be used for this purpose. However, compliance rates remain low and cost-effectiveness is questionable.
- Medical management for UUI includes anticholinergic and nonanticholinergic medications, the efficacy and safety of which have been demonstrated (**Table 5.3**).[2] Overall continuation rates range from 40% to 58% at 3 months to 17% to 35% at 12 months.
- For overactive bladder, posterior tibial nerve stimulation (PTNS) involves placement of a single thin acupuncture-type needle at the posterior distal tibial nerve for the treatment of UUI (**Figure 5.1**). Stimulation through a portable pulse generator is applied to the needle for a series of 12 30-minute weekly sessions. Akin to acupuncture, the therapy is office based and has minimal adverse effects. Outcomes are similar to that of anticholinergic medication.[3]

IMAGING AND OTHER DIAGNOSTICS

- Diagnostic evaluation may be used when additional information might impact patient counseling and treatment planning. For example, in cases where initial history and examination are inconsistent or inconclusive and a clear diagnosis is not obtained. Other indications for further evaluation include mixed UI, overactive bladder (OAB) symptoms, prior surgery, neurogenic bladder, abnormal initial evaluation, severe concomitant pelvic organ prolapse, or voiding dysfunction.[1]

Table 5.3 Medical Management of UUI

Medication, Generic (Brand)	Dosage
Darifenacin (Enablex ER)	7.5–15 mg by mouth daily
Fesoterodine (Toviaz)	4–8 mg by mouth daily
Solifenacin (Vesicare)	5–10 mg by mouth daily
Mirabegron (Myrbetriq ER)	25–50 mg by mouth daily
Oxybutynin (Ditropan)	5 mg by mouth one to three times daily
Oxybutynin (Ditropan XL)	5–15 mg by mouth daily
Oxybutynin topical (Gelnique)	84–100 mg transdermal daily
Oxybutynin topical (Oxytrol)	1 patch transdermal changed twice per week
Tolterodine (Detrol)	1–2 mg by mouth twice daily
Tolterodine (Detrol LA)	2–4 mg by mouth daily
Trospium (Sanctura)	20 mg by mouth twice daily
Trospium (Sanctura ER)	60 mg by mouth daily

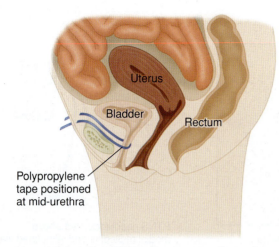

Figure 5.2. Mid-urethral sling placement under midportion of urethra.

- Further diagnostics are not required when treating patients with uncomplicated, straightforward SUI considering surgery.[4]
- Diagnostic evaluation may include one or more of the following:
  - A bladder diary or frequency–volume chart, is a record of liquid intake, urinary output, and UI of at least one consecutive 24-hour period. This information can be helpful to establish an objective baseline and for the clinician to understand exacerbating factors, symptom severity, and impact on activities of daily living.
  - Pad weight tests may be used to quantify UI. Duration of testing ranges in practice from 1 to 48 hours.
  - Urodynamics refers to an interactive series of tests used to evaluate bladder filling, storage, and emptying. Tests may include PVR, cystometry, uroflowmetry, and pressure flow studies. Supplemental modalities of video (x-ray) studies, electromyography, and/or urethral function tests may be added. Urodynamics should be selectively performed in patients considering surgical management of UI.

PREOPERATIVE PLANNING

- The goal of all UI treatments is to reduce incontinence episodes and improve quality of life. Preoperative planning begins with an overall assessment of the patient's reported symptoms, objective findings, and most importantly, treatment goals. Understanding of risks, benefits, and treatment alternatives as well as physical capacity to manage unexpected outcomes is essential.
- Cystoscopy under local anesthesia may be considered prior to surgical management of UI to evaluate for other causes (see Chapter 10: Cystoscopy).

- For patients with SUI, consider:
  - Documenting attempts at nonsurgical management such as behavior modification and PFME prior to surgical management.
  - Consideration of age, activity level, and need for possible repeat treatment when considering surgical treatment options.
  - Informed consent regarding the safety and efficacy of synthetic or biologic material used for this purpose, including possible short- and long-term complications.
  - Physical ability to use indwelling or clean intermittent catheters in cases of postoperative urinary retention.
- A **mid-urethral sling** (MUS) is the mainstay for surgical management of SUI (Fig. 5.2). A MUS should be considered in these scenarios:
  - Strongly desire durable long-term outcomes
  - Bothersome SUI with activity, exertion (cough, laugh, sneeze)
  - Vaginally parous women
  - Hypermobile urethra
  - Understands and consents to use of permanent synthetic mesh
- **Pubovaginal sling** (Fig. 5.3) should be strongly considered in scenarios similar to an MUS but in women who are poor candidates or are averse to the use of a synthetic material.
  - Prior unsuccessful mid-urethral synthetic sling procedure
- **Transurethral bulking** (Fig. 5.4) should be strongly considered in these scenarios:
  - SUI without prior vaginal delivery
  - Nonmobile urethra

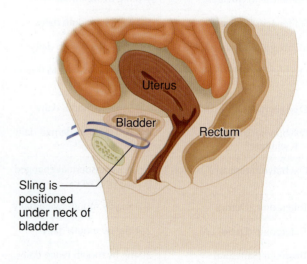

Figure 5.3. Pubovaginal sling placement under proximal portion of urethra or bladder neck.

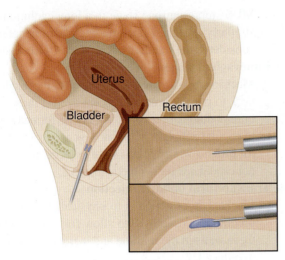

Figure 5.4. Transurethral bulking of material into suburothelium.

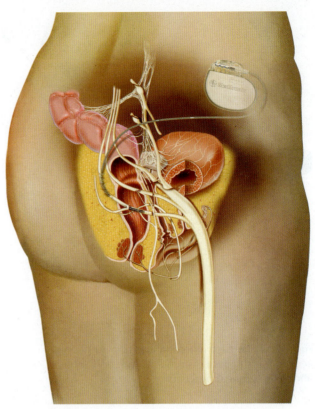

Figure 5.5. Sacral neuromodulation or sacral nerve stimulation involves the placement of electrodes under fluoroscopic guidance for stimulation of the S2, S3, and S4 nerve roots via their foramina. (From Jones HW, Rock JA. *Te Linde's Operative Gynecology*. 11th ed. Philadelphia, PA: Wolters Kluwer; 2015. Image provided by Medtronic, Inc.)

- Intrinsic sphincter deficiency
- Bothersome mild SUI with activity
- Poor operative candidate
- Prior anti-incontinence procedure, particularly failed or complicated slings
- For patients with UUI, consider:
  - Documenting lack of efficacy of nonsurgical management such as bladder retraining or medications
  - Consideration of age, activity level, physical capability, and need for possible repeat treatment when considering surgical treatment options
  - Informed consent regarding the safety and efficacy of permanently implanted foreign bodies used for this purpose, including possible short- and long-term complications
- **Cystoscopic injection** with botulinum toxin, a treatment for overactive bladder or urge incontinence should be strongly considered in these scenarios:
  - Bothersome daily UUI
  - Demonstrated detrusor contractions
  - Accepts need for repeat treatment as efficacy decreases with time
  - Physical ability to use indwelling or clean intermittent catheters
- **Sacral neuromodulation** (Fig. 5.5) should be strongly considered in these scenarios:
  - Bothersome overactive bladder or UUI daily
  - Demonstrated detrusor contractions
  - Success with other forms of neuromodulation
  - Physical ability to manage device and programming
  - Strongly desire durable long-term outcomes
  - Understanding that the pulse generator may limit the use of one's ability to undergo magnetic resonance imaging (MRI)

SURGICAL MANAGEMENT

- Surgical management is available for SUI and UUI. Perioperative risks are generally low similar to other benign gynecologic surgery and most procedures can be performed with minimal or no anesthesia.
- All procedures should be performed in rooms of sufficient size to allow for the surgeon and assistant as well as cystoscopy equipment.
- Urinary infection should be ruled out and PVR should be documented prior to UI procedures.

Positioning

- UI procedures are performed with the patient in lithotomy position similar to other gynecologic procedures. MUSs, pubovaginal slings, and cystoscopic procedures are performed with the patient in lithotomy (Fig. 5.6).
  - Various lithotomy stirrups are available to assure patient safety and comfort, minimizing risk for related peripheral neuropathic injury.
- Sacral neuromodulation is performed with the patient in prone position with additional support.

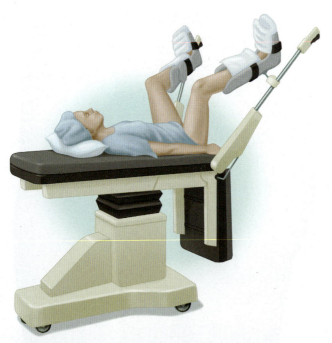

Figure 5.6. Standard lithotomy position for perineal access, transurethral instrumentation, or combined abdominoperineal procedures.

- The chest is supported laterally with rolled blankets or pillows for comfortable breathing during the procedure.
- The hips are similarly supported so that the pelvis is elevated, flat, and parallel with the floor.
- The feet are similarly supported and accessible to assistants during the procedure.

Approach

- Surgical treatment for UI can be performed in a minimally invasive fashion, in an outpatient setting using local anesthesia with intravenous sedation, regional, or general anesthesia.
  - **Mid-urethral slings**
    - Mechanism of action is to support the urethra and bladder neck in a hammock shape to provide elevation, support, and at times, partial compression. MUSs represent one stage in a long evolution of similarly designed operations and are generally considered the standard of care for SUI treatment.
  - **Pubovaginal slings**
    - Mechanism of action is to support the bladder neck to prevent urethral descent against increased intra-abdominal pressure. Widely performed prior to popularization of MUSs now generally reserved for patients whose MUSs were unsuccessful or are not candidates for synthetic material.
  - **Transurethral bulking injection**
    - Mechanism of action is to physically bolster the urethral mucosal layer to allow for coaptation of these walls in the midline and increase resistance to reduce UI.
    - Can be performed using mild sedation and local anesthesia alone and therefore an excellent choice for women with medical comorbidities, extreme elderly, or cannot tolerate general anesthesia or in whom immobility should be avoided.
- The approach to the surgical management of **UUI** should focus on overall impact of symptoms on quality of life. Assessment of bother due to urinary symptoms together with quantifying episodes is essential to the discussion of treatment options. Clear understanding of treatment goals and expectations will improve patient satisfaction. Patients who fail initial behavioral and medical management can be counseled for cystoscopic injection of onabotulinum toxin A or sacral neuromodulation as both treatments can be performed using minimal or no anesthesia in the office or outpatient surgery setting.
  - **Cystoscopic injection** of botulinum toxin
    - Mechanism of action is local denervation of the detrusor muscle by onabotulinum toxin (Botox, Allergan).
  - **Sacral neuromodulation**
    - Mechanism of action is to restore balance to the neuromuscular control of the detrusor muscle. Exact mechanism remains unknown.
- There is no consensus on the treatment of recurrent SUI following MUS.[5]

Mid-Urethral Slings (Tech Fig. 5.1)

- In mid-urethral slings (MUSs), the central portion of the hammock is placed under the mid-urethra between the urethra and vaginal wall. In addition to the retropubic route, transobturator, prepubic, and infrapelvic single incision routes have been described. Comparative data support retropubic and transobturator as most efficacious techniques.
- MUSs may be fashioned from synthetic or biologic material; however the term generally refers to synthetic slings.[6]

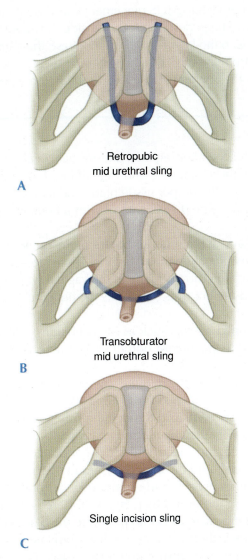

Tech Figure 5.1. Examples of sling placement. **A:** Retropubic sling. **B:** Transobturator sling. **C:** Single incision sling. (Modified from Wound, Ostomy and Continence Nurses Society®, Doughty DB, Moore KN. *Wound, Ostomy and Continence Nurses Society® Core Curriculum: Continence Management*. Philadelphia, PA: Wolters Kluwer; 2015; Kovac RS, Zimmerman CS. *Advances in Reconstructive Vaginal Surgery*. 2nd ed. Philadelphia, PA: Lippincott Williams & Wilkins; 2012.)

- The use of synthetic material for sling procedures has evolved since its introduction. Mersilene slings were described by Williams and Te Linde in 1962 and later replaced by silicone but both materials were associated with pain, erosions, and infections. Marlex, nylon, silastic, and Gore-Tex slings have also been described. Polypropylene has remained the most commonly used synthetic material for MUSs since 1996 due to its relative safety compared to antecedent synthetic materials.[11]
- MUSs can be placed using a retropubic or transobturator approach. This refers to the route of passage of the sling arms in contrast to the midportion which lies at the mid-urethra.
  - Retropubic approach to MUS placement was first described with the tension-free vaginal tape (TVT) procedure by Ulmsten[11] in 1996 and long-term outcomes were also reported. This procedure has served as the comparison for the development of subsequent slings. Variations of surgical placement have been described. The "top-down" approach refers to passage of trocars from the retropubic space to the vagina. In contrast, the "bottom-up" approach refers to passage of trocars from the vagina to the retropubic space.
  - Transobturator (TO) approach to MUS placement was described in 2001. Variations of surgical placement have been described. The "inside-out" approach refers to passage of trocars from the vagina to the lateral thighs. In contrast, the "outside-in" approach refers to passage of trocars from the thighs to the vagina.
- The patient is placed on the operating table in dorsal lithotomy position.

Retropubic Approach

- Typically performed with general or regional anesthesia. Local anesthetic may be injected into the skin at the site of the suprapubic and vaginal incisions. Injection of larger volumes is often used to hydrodissect the proper tissue plane and facilitate entry. Commonly used preparations include bupivacaine 0.25% with or without epinephrine, dilute vasopressin, and normal saline 0.9%.
- Two stab incisions are made at the superior border of the pubic symphysis approximately 6 cm apart centered across the abdominal midline. These represent the final location of the sling arms. A single vertical incision is made in the vaginal wall approximately 1.5 cm long at the location of the mid-urethra. This represents the final location of the sling midportion (see **Pearls and Pitfalls**).
- Using a sharp, narrow-tipped scissors such as Metzenbaums, a tunnel is created under the vaginal wall laterally toward the inferior border of the pubic symphysis. This is repeated on the contralateral side (Tech Fig. 5.2).
- The trocar arm is inserted through the midline vaginal incision and slid into the previously dissected tunnel with the sling attached (Tech Fig. 5.3).
- A straight catheter guide may be placed through the Foley catheter into the bladder to deviate the bladder away from the trocar during passage.
- The trocar is then advanced: the levator muscle is perforated entering the space of Retzius. The trocar handle should be angled toward the floor bringing the tip of the trocar up along the posterior aspect of the symphysis, perforate the rectus fascia, and out through the preformed skin incisions (Tech Fig. 5.4). Care is taken to maintain the angle and carefully control the trocar so as not to perforate the bladder medially or bowel proximally. The procedure is then repeated on the contralateral side. The sling is now in place, cystoscopy is performed to ensure no transgression. Once confirmed tensioning can take place.

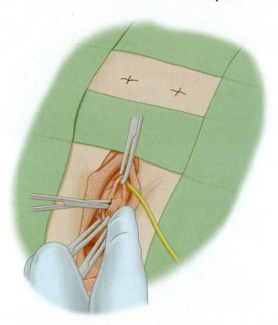

Tech Figure 5.2. Retropubic sling incisions. Two stab incisions are made at the superior border of the pubic symphysis approximately 3 to 6 cm apart centered across the abdominal midline. A single vertical incision is made in the vaginal wall approximately 1.5 cm long at the location of the mid-urethra. A tunnel is created under the vaginal wall laterally toward the inferior border of the pubic symphysis.

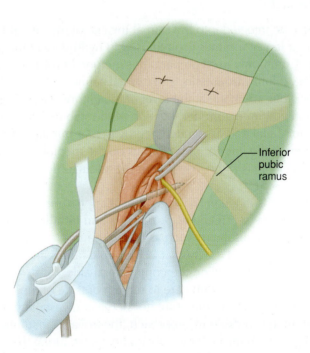

Tech Figure 5.3. Retropubic sling placement of trocar. The trocar arm is inserted through the midline vaginal incision and slid into the previously dissected tunnel with the sling attached.

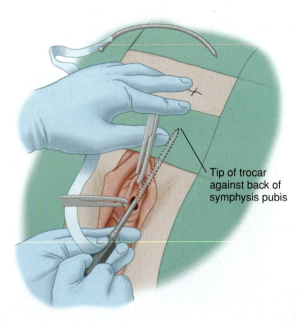

Tech Figure 5.4. Retropubic sling passing trocar. The trocar is advanced traversing the perineal membrane. The trocar handle should be angled toward the floor bringing the tip of the trocar up to advance immediately against the posterior aspect of the symphysis, then perforating the rectus fascia and coming out through the skin incisions.

Transobturator Approach

- Local anesthetic may be injected into the skin at the site of the lateral thigh and vaginal incisions. Injection of larger volumes is often used to hydrodissect the proper tissue plane and facilitate entry. Commonly used preparations include bupivacaine 0.25% with or without epinephrine, dilute vasopressin, and normal saline 0.9%.
- Two lateral stab incisions are made at the level of the clitoris. Palpation of the obturator foramen can assist in confirming proper location of the stab incisions. A safe starting point to avoid the obturator canal and associated neurovascular bundle is to place incisions right along the border of the inferior pubic ramus on the medial margin of the obturator foramen. This is typically below the insertion of the adductor longus and just lateral to the gluteal folds (**Tech Fig. 5.5**).
- A single vertical incision is made in the vaginal wall approximately 1.5 cm long at the location of the mid-urethra (see **Tech Fig. 5.6**; **Pearls and Pitfalls**).
- Using a sharp, narrow-tipped scissors such as Metzenbaums, a tunnel is created under the vaginal wall laterally toward the medial ischiopubic ramus and inferior border of the obturator foramen. This is repeated on the contralateral side.
- The trocar is guided horizontally, with care to remain outside of the endopelvic fascia and peritoneal cavity, and not to injure the obturator nerve and vasculature transiting through the obturator canal. In the "outside-in" approach, the trocar is first introduced through the skin incision. Passage is then through the subcutaneous fat, along the adductor muscles, through the inferior border of the obturator foramen followed by the obturator internus and levator ani muscles. The trocar tip is then guided through into the vagina at the previously made incision at the mid-urethra. The sling is attached to the trocar tip and the trocar is then gently reversed back through the groin incision, pulling the sling into position. The procedure is then repeated on the contralateral side.

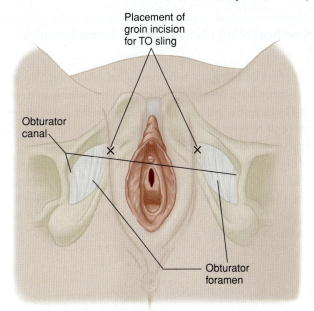

Tech Figure 5.5. Obturator foramen anatomy. Obturator canal containing artery and nerve is located on ventral lateral margin of obturator foramen. Incisions should be placed on the medial aspect of the obturator foramen at the level of clitoris. TO = transobturator.

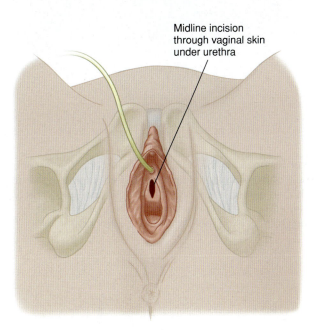

Tech Figure 5.6. Midline suburethral incision. A single vertical incision is made in the vaginal wall, approximately 1.5 cm long, at the location of the mid-urethra.

Once the sling has been passed, cystoscopy is performed to confirm no bladder or urethral perforation has occurred (see **Pearls and Pitfalls**). In rare cases of perforation, the trocars are removed and replaced in a similar manner. Closure of the cystotomy puncture site is not necessary. If the urethra has been injured during placement, the urethra should be repaired and the sling NOT placed.

Tensioning of Mid-Urethral Sling (Retropubic or Transobturator)
(Tech Figs. 5.7 and 5.9)

- After confirmation of bladder integrity, tensioning is performed. Notably, there is no single accepted way of accomplishing proper tensioning. Key principle in tensioning is to be "tension free" (Tech Fig. 5.8). Avoid elevation of the urethra and err on the side of leaving sling loose to obviate risk of retention. Various approaches have been described. Below are some of the commonly performed techniques:
  - Holding excess sling material through the midline incision using a Babcock clamp. Leaving a small "knuckle" of mesh. This method capitalizes on the normal deformation of the mesh during placement and will "shrink" once in situ (Tech Fig. 5.9).
  - Placing a large scissor or right angle clamp under the urethra with space between the mesh and urethra (Tech Fig. 5.10).

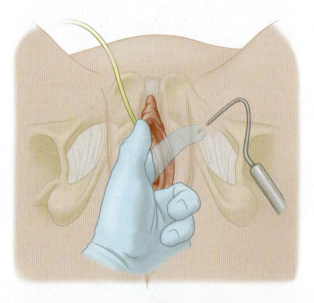

Tech Figure 5.7. Insertion of TO trocar. In the "outside-in" approach, the trocar is first introduced through the skin incision. The fascia of the obturator externus and then muscle of the obturator internus are traversed. The trocar tip is then guided by the surgeon's finger out through the vagina at the previously made incision at the mid-urethra. The sling is attached to the trocar tip and the trocar is then gently reversed back through the groin incision, pulling the sling into position.

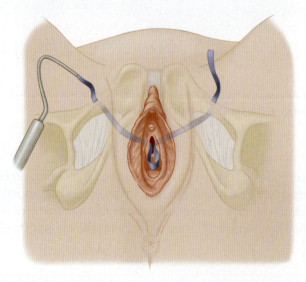

Tech Figure 5.8. TO mesh sling in situ. After both sides of the sling are placed, the sling is ready for tensioning.

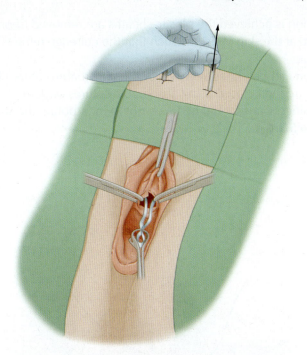

Tech Figure 5.9. Mid-urethral sling tensioning with Babcock. Using a Babcock clamp to grasp a small "knuckle" of mesh will allow adequate tensioning.

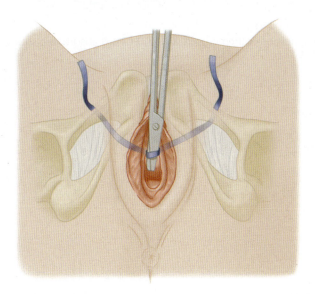

Tech Figure 5.10. Mid-urethral sling tensioning with scissor. Using a large scissor or right angle clamp to maintain space between the urethra and mesh during sheath removal will allow for adequate tensioning.

- Once desired tension is achieved the plastic sheaths are removed (if present) and excess material is trimmed at the skin incisions such that the cut edge retracts beneath the subcutaneous tissue.
- The vaginal incision can be closed with 3.0 or 4.0 absorbable suture (Tech Fig. 5.11).
- The skin incisions are then closed using absorbable sutures or dermal adhesive and covered with dressings. Care should be taken not to incorporate the sling material into the skin closure (Video 5.1).

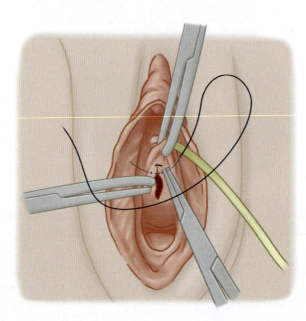

Tech Figure 5.11. Vaginal incision is then closed with 3.0 or 4.0 absorbable suture.

Pubovaginal Slings

- In a pubovaginal sling, the central portion of the hammock is traditionally placed more proximally under the bladder neck between the bladder and the vaginal wall. This in contrast to the MUSs described above.
- Pubovaginal slings may be of synthetic or biologic material but the term traditionally refers to a sling fashioned from biologic material.
    - Biologic material includes autografts, allografts, or xenografts. Autologous grafts involve harvest of rectus fascia or fascia lata. Allografts and xenografts may originate from fascia, dermis, bladder, or other organ material.

Pubovaginal Sling Approach

- Local anesthetic may be injected into the skin at the site of the suprapubic and vaginal incisions. Injection of larger volumes is often used to hydrodissect the proper tissue plane and facilitate entry. Commonly used preparations include bupivacaine 0.25% with or without epinephrine, dilute vasopressin, and normal saline 0.9%.
- A transverse suprapubic stab incision is made 2 cm superior to the pubic symphysis and 2 to 4 cm in length. Vaginal incisions can be performed in one of two fashions, always with care taken only to incise the wall and not to penetrate the periurethral fascia:
    - A single vertical incision in the vaginal wall approximately 2 to 3 cm long at the location of the bladder neck. In this approach, the sling tunnel is created by dissecting laterally.
    - Two lateral incisions in the vaginal wall approximately 1.5 cm long at the location of the bladder neck. In this approach, the sling tunnel is created by dissecting under the epithelium across the midline to connect the incisions.
- Using a sharp, narrow-tipped scissors such as Metzenbaums, a tunnel is created under the vaginal wall lateral to the bladder neck, to the inferior aspect of the pubic symphysis. The tip of blunt scissors such as Mayo scissors are placed parallel to the symphysis at the posteroinferior border with tips aimed away from the bladder. Using gentle pressure the scissors are slid along the symphysis and the urethropelvic ligament and the endopelvic fascia is perforated to enter the retropubic space. Finger palpation confirms entry. This is repeated on the contralateral side.
- A sling is then fashioned using the graft for the midportion of the sling and then attaching sutures to the lateral margins of the sling for the carriage arms.
    - Size is approximately 1.5 cm in width and 12 to 14 cm in length such that there is sufficient length that it will pass posterior to the symphysis and scar in place, approximating the natural position of the pubourethral ligament.
    - Commonly used suture arm materials include absorbable suture such as Vicryl (polyglactin 910, Ethicon Johnson & Johnson, Somerville, NJ) or nonabsorbable suture such as Prolene (polypropylene or polydioxanone [PDS], Ethicon Johnson & Johnson, Somerville, NJ). One suture with two tails is attached to each side of the sling and should be at least 12 cm in length to allow for passage without tension (Tech Fig. 5.12).
- A double-pronged needle carrier is used to pass the sling. For example, the Pereyra-Raz carrier (Tech Fig. 5.13; Cook Urological Inc., Spencer, IN). The tips of the carrier are inserted though the suprapubic incision and subcutaneous fat, perforating the rectus fascia, and entering the previously created retropubic tunnel.

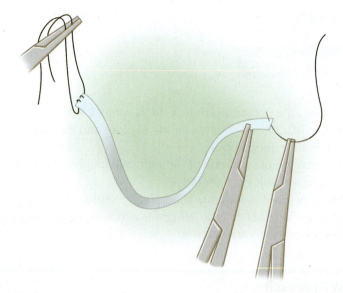

Tech Figure 5.12. Biologic sling.

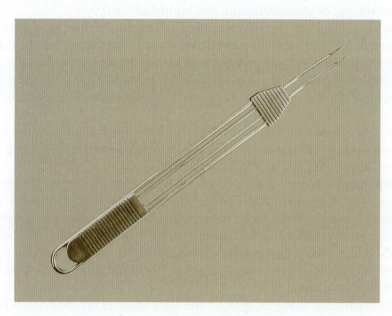

Tech Figure 5.13. Pereyra-Raz ligature carrier. (Courtesy of Cook Urological Inc., Spencer, IN.)

- Using the surgeon's nondominant hand, the index finger is placed in the retropubic tunnel through the vaginal incision. The needle carrier tip is then met by the surgeon's vaginal finger prior to rectus fascial perforation, and the tip gently guided out through the vaginal incision under control. This ensures the carrier tips do not perforate the bladder, bladder neck, or urethra in its path.
- Each arm of the sling suture is then fed through an eye of the needle passer with only a small tail remaining. The passer is then gently guided in reverse, leading the sling through the tunnel and out through the suprapubic incision. This is repeated on the contralateral side (Tech Fig. 5.14).
- Passage of the sling across the bladder neck is accomplished depending on the type of incision made.
  - In cases of midline incision, the sling can simply be gently laid across the mid-urethral after passage of the first arm through the suprapubic incision.
  - In cases of lateral entry, the sling must be passed through the tunnel prior to passage of the second arm through the suprapubic incision. This can be accomplished by using a grasping clamp such as a tonsil through the contralateral incision, across the tunnel, to exit on the side where the sling is located. The free sutures are grasped with the clamp, which is then gently slid in reverse such that the sling is gently pulled into position through the tunnel. The arm is then ready for placement in the ipsilateral suprapubic tunnel.

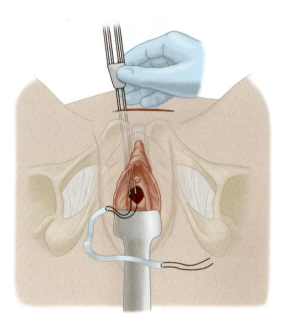
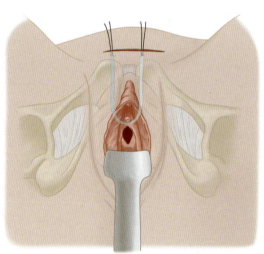

Tech Figure 5.14. Pubovaginal sling procedure. A transverse strip of autologous fascia has been harvested from the transverse abdominal incision or separately from fascia lata on the leg. An incision in the vagina under the proximal urethral allows a finger dissection into the retropubic space so that the ligature carrier can be passed from the abdominal incision under continuous and direct guidance. The permanent sutures attached to the sling are brought through the carrier and brought up through the abdominal incision, and the sling is secured to the rectus fascia. (Adapted from an illustration by J. Tan-Kim, MD. In: Gibbs RS, Karlan BY, Haney AF, Nygaard IE. *Danforth's Obstetrics and Gynecology*. 10th ed. Philadelphia, PA: Wolters Kluwer; 2008.)

- Once the sling has been passed, cystoscopy is performed to confirm no bladder perforation has occurred.
- In cases of bladder perforation, the sutures are backed away and replaced in a similar manner. Closure of the cystotomy puncture site is not necessary, however bladder drainage should be performed postoperatively for 3 to 7 days.
- After confirmation of bladder integrity the sling can be sutured to the perivesical tissue on either side of the midline with 3.0 plain gut suture to prevent migration or rolling.
- The sutures can be tied down ipsilaterally when a double-pronged passer is used. If single-pronged passer is used, then tying the sutures across the midline fascial bridge is necessitated.
- Tension is set to allow a heavy scissor or right angle clamp between the sling and urethra.
- The skin incisions are then closed using absorbable sutures or skin adhesive and covered with dressings.

Transurethral Bulking

- The term "transurethral" refers to delivery method. The procedure is performed via operative cystoscopy under direct visualization generally in ambulatory surgical setting. The patient is placed in lithotomy position to administer local anesthetic. Lidocaine gel may be used for the urethra and this is most often sufficient for pain relief during the procedure. Sedation may be used for patients who are unable to tolerate the procedure using local anesthesia alone.
- During this time the medication should be prepared for injection.
  - Multiple bulking agents are commercially available. Materials used over the years have included autologous tissue, silicone, collagen, calcium hydroxylapatite, ethylene vinyl alcohol, carbon spheres, polydimethylsiloxane, and dextranomer hyaluronic acid. Though there is insufficient evidence to recommend one agent over another, current practice patterns demonstrate polydimethylsiloxane and calcium hydroxylapatite are the two most commonly used.[7]
  - Endoscopic needles or customized devices are used for injection. Many are commercially available and some are specific to implant type. A syringe with bulking material is attached to the cystoscopic needle or customized device as instructed.
- Cystoscopy is then performed using a 12- or 30-degree lens and distending fluid.
  - Diagnostic cystoscopy should be performed if not done previously. Assessment of detrusor muscle and visualization of anatomic abnormalities are documented.
  - The cystoscope is then withdrawn to the mid-urethra until the level of the urethral sphincter is visualized. The injection sites used for coaptite are the 4 and 8 o'clock positions for injections recommending two sites, and 2, 10, and 6 o'clock for those agents recommending three distinct sites.
  - The cystoscope is then angled approximately 45 degrees toward the urethra and the needle advanced to puncture the mucosa. The needle tip should be just beneath the mucosal surface. The cystoscope is then angled back toward midline to be parallel with the urethra. This ensures the needle tip is in a tunnel parallel to the urethral axis (see **Tech Fig. 5.15**).

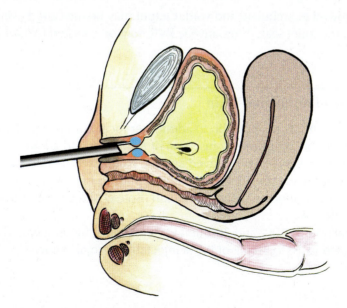

Tech Figure 5.15. Transurethral bulking. Under cystoscopic visualization, a transurethral needle injects a bulking agent into multiple submucosal sites in the proximal urethra to increase urethral resistance. (Illustration by J. Tan-Kim, MD. In: Gibbs RS, Karlan BY, Haney AF, Nygaard IE. *Danforth's Obstetrics and Gynecology*. 10th ed. Philadelphia, PA: Wolters Kluwer; 2008.)

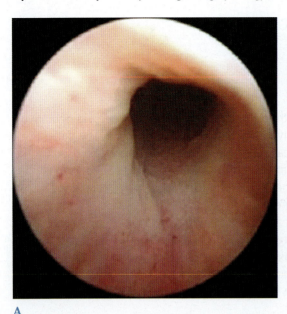 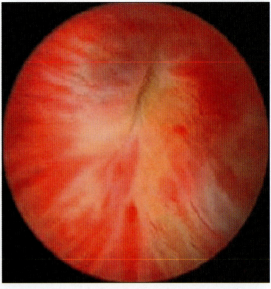

A B

Tech Figure 5.16. Pre- and postinjection state of the urethral sphincter. **A:** Preinjection state. The urethral lumen is wide open. **B:** Postinjection state. The urethral lumen is coaptated. (From Lee SW, Kang JH, Sung HH, et al. Treatment outcomes of transurethral macroplastique injection for postprostatectomy incontinence. *Korean J Urol.* 2014;55[3]:182–189.)

- The material is then injected under direct visualization. The mucosal layer should appear to fill circumferentially toward the midline. Once the mucosa is at the midline, the needle is withdrawn.
- The procedure is repeated at the remaining sites until adequate urethral coaptation is appreciated (Tech Fig. 5.16).
- Following injection the bladder may be emptied and refilled with 200 to 300 cc of normal saline. The cystoscope is removed and the patient returned to supine position.
- The patient is allowed to ambulate and void. Output may be measured using a hat placed under the toilet seat. Alternatively, PVR may be checked following this void.

Cystoscopic Injection of Botulinum Toxin

- The patient is placed in lithotomy position to administer local anesthetic. Lidocaine gel may be used for the urethra, followed by insertion of a catheter and administration of 30 cc of 2% lidocaine. The catheter is then removed and the patient returned to supine position. The medication may optimally remain for 30 minutes prior to initiation of procedure.
- During this time the medication onabotulinum toxin (Botox, Allergan) should be prepared for injection (see Table 5.4).
  - Medication is available in 100- and 200-unit vials and must be refrigerated until usage. It is typically diluted in 10 to 30 mL of 0.9% injectable normal saline.

Table 5.4	Onabotulinum Toxin Dosage and Urinary Retention Risk[9,10]
Dosage (Units)	Urinary Retention Risk (%)
50	9
100	18
150	25
200	25
300	25

- Cystoscopy is then performed using a 12- or 30-degree lens and normal saline for irrigation fluid.
  - The anesthetic solution should be drained and bladder rinsed. Diagnostic cystoscopy may be performed if not done previously. Assessment of detrusor muscle and visualization of anatomic abnormalities are documented.
  - Cystoscopic needles are used for medication injection. Many are commercially available. Typical sizes are 22- to 23-gauge, 3- to 7-French width, 2- to 8-mL needle tip length.
  - A syringe with the medication is attached to the cystoscopic needle. Medication is administered into the detrusor muscle under direct visualization in 5- to 10-unit increments (0.5- to 1-cc injection volume). In general, injections are placed in multiple quadrants so that the medication is equally distributed across the detrusor muscle (Tech Fig. 5.17).
  - Following injection the bladder may be emptied. The cystoscope is removed and the patient returned to supine position.
  - Postprocedural care should be implemented with follow-up residual urine in 10 to 14 days.

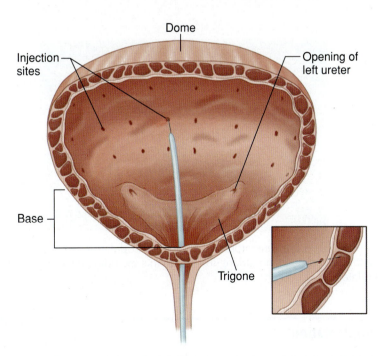

Tech Figure 5.17. Injection of botulinum toxin for the treatment of urinary urge incontinence and overactive bladder. (Modified from Nitti VW. Botulinum toxin for the treatment of idiopathic and neurogenic overactive bladder: State of the art. *Rev Urol.* 2006;8[4]:198–208.)

Sacral Neuromodulation

- Sacral neuromodulation is approved for the treatment of refractory urge UI, urgency-frequency, nonobstructive urinary retention, and fecal incontinence and is used off-label for pelvic pain since 1997 and 1999. Since first described by the anterior approach in 1976 by Brindley and colleagues, sacral neuromodulation technique has evolved to the current method of a posterior approach to the S3 nerve roots with or without fluoroscopic guidance for the treatment of urologic disorders (see **Pearls and Pitfalls**).
- The current technique involves two stages. First, a test stage wherein the patient trials sacral neuromodulation for a few days up to 4 weeks to determine whether or not there is treatment benefit. Subjective improvement and/or objective improvement of ≥50% are generally considered benefit. Second, an implantation stage wherein the successful patients undergo implantation of the implantable pulse generator (IPG) (**Tech Fig. 5.18**). Those whose trials were unsuccessful undergo complete removal of test stage components.

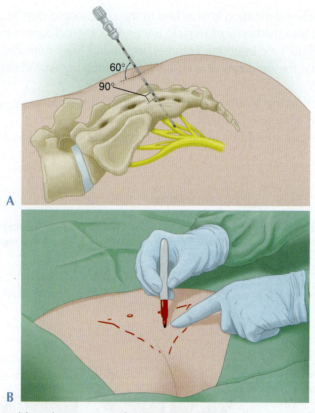

Tech Figure 5.18. Implantable pulse generator for sacral neuromodulation. **A:** Angle of the insertion needle penetrating the sacrum **B:** Skin marking the landmarks including the coccyx in the midline and the ischial spines bilaterally.

Percutaneous Implantation

Percutaneous implantation refers to a technique by which a percutaneous nerve evaluation (PNE) is performed in the first stage (testing phase), and the final electrode and IPG are placed in the second stage. The first stage can be performed in an office setting under local anesthetic.

Staged Implantation

- Staged implantation refers to a technique by which the final electrode (Tech Fig. 5.19) is placed in the first stage (testing phase) and the IPG is attached in the second stage.
- Staged implantation is performed in an ambulatory surgical setting under sedation with local anesthetic.
- The outpatient nature of this procedure makes sacral neuromodulation an excellent option for patients in whom general anesthesia poses significant risks. Though the motor response is most critical the avoidance of general anesthesia allows for intraoperative sensory feedback which can facilitate optimal lead placement.

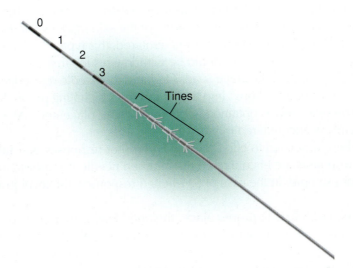

Tech Figure 5.19. Tined electrode for final placement for sacral neuromodulation. Each lead has four electrodes (0–3).

Staged Implantation: First Stage

- After proper positioning and patient comfort are confirmed, surgical draping can be performed. Caution is taken to maintain a sterile field as contamination of foreign bodies designed for permanent implantation may increase the risk of infection and the need for explantation of infected material.
    - The surgical field should include the lower back, sacrum, buttocks, and anus. Use of Ioban (3M, St. Paul, MN) is recommended.
    - The buttocks may be taped laterally such that the anus is visible to the surgeon during the procedure.
    - Feet should be visible to the surgeon during the procedure and accessible to assistants outside the sterile field.
- Identification of the S3 foramina is then performed. This can be accomplished with or without fluoroscopy:
    - The coccyx is palpated. A ruler is used to measure 9 cm cranially in the midline. A line is drawn at this level perpendicular to the spine to identify the approximate location of S3 (Tech Fig 5.18B). The medial aspect of the foramen is approximately 2 cm from the spinal midline. This distance can similarly be measured with a ruler and marked parallel to the spine. The intersection of these lines approximates the proper location for lead placement.
    - Landmarks can also be identified using fluoroscopy. The patient must be on a surgical table that allows for C-arm rotation below the pelvis. An anterior-posterior (AP) view is

obtained to identify the medial border of the foramen and a marking is made parallel to the midline. A lateral view is then obtained and the curvature of the sacroiliac joint is identified, which is the approximate location of S2. The next caudal level is S3. A radiopaque marker such as a clamp or wire can be used to properly identify S3 and the loban is then marked.

- The skin is then infiltrated with local anesthesia, most commonly either lidocaine or bupivacaine. The innervated areas that are associated with the most procedural discomfort are the periosteum and the skin. We suggest infiltration of 1 to 2 cc at the level of the periosteum followed by skin infiltration. The subcutaneous tissue need not be infiltrated significantly.
- The foramen needle is then inserted into S3 using the identified landmarks. Generally, the needle should follow cephalad to caudal pathway and from medial to lateral to approximate the pathway of the S3 nerves as they exit and travel along the anterior sacrum.
  - The tip is inserted at the approximate location of the skin markers parallel to the path of the S3 canal (**Fig 5.18A**). If resistance is encountered, this typically signals the periosteum has been reached and the needle should be withdrawn such that the tip remains just below the skin level, then the angle is adjusted and the needle reinserted. This process is repeated until the needle "drops" into the S3 foramen, signaling proper location.
  - Lateral fluoroscopic view is obtained to confirm proper placement. AP view can also be used if difficulty is encountered in intubating the foramen.
- The needle is then stimulated to elicit sensory and motor responses (see **Table 5.5**). If S2 or S4 level responses are encountered the foramen needle is removed and adjusted accordingly. For example, in the case of S2 elicited responses, the level just caudad should be intubated.
- Once the foramen needle is in proper place, the tined lead is then placed.
  - The skin is incised approximately 1 cm at the location of the foramen needle.
  - The stylet is then grasped and removed from the foramen needle. A ¼ turn counterclockwise may be necessary to free the stylet.
  - A guidewire is placed through the foramen needle and gently guided to be past the level of the anterior sacrum. Lateral fluoroscopic view may be obtained.
  - The foramen needle is then gently guided out and off the guidewire, with care to ensure the guidewire does not become dislodged.
  - The T-shaped introducer sheath is then inserted. The guidewire is fed through the central canal, then the sheath guided down through the skin toward the anterior sacrum along the path of the wire. Care should be taken to make sure the wire is not bent during this portion of the procedure. The radiopaque tip of the sheath should be approximately at the anterior border of the sacrum on lateral fluoroscopic view.
  - The guidewire is then gently removed from the introducer sheath.
  - The introducer is then removed from the sheath. A ¼ turn clockwise of the introducer should release it from the sheath and then it can be guided outward.
  - The tined lead is then inserted through the sheath, with care not to bend it at this portion of the procedure. A white radiopaque marker denotes the proper depth of the lead and

Table 5.5 Sacral Nerve Sensory and Motor Responses

Nerve	Sensory Response	Motor Response
S2	Vagina	Foot dorsiflexion, heel rotation Anal sphincter contraction
S3	Vagina, perineum, rectum	Great toe dorsiflexion Bellows[a]
S4	Rectum, anus	Bellows[a]

[a]Inward pull of the gluteus and anus.

should be at the top of the sheath. Lateral fluoroscopic view will reveal the electrodes (e.g., four in a quadripolar lead) whose location should follow the natural path of the nerve. Most commonly, electrodes 0 and 1 are anterior to the sacrum, and electrodes 2 and 3 straddle the anterior border of the sacrum.

- At this juncture, the electrodes can be stimulated to elicit sensory and motor responses. A nonsterile surgical assistant is typically required. The lead can be gently adjusted anterior or posterior until sufficient responses are generated in the majority of electrodes. This stage is of the upmost importance as proper placement will ensure the maximum possibilities for programming the device postoperatively.
- Once proper location is confirmed, the sheath is gently removed along the lead with caution taken not to dislodge the lead with fluoroscopy assistance.
- Fluoroscopic views of lead location should be taken and stored for the medical record. In the lateral view, the lead should appear straight through the sacrum and then deviate slightly caudally. In AP view, the lead should follow medial to lateral pathway and appear similar to a hockey stick with a gentle curve following the natural anatomic course of the nerves.
- The lead is then tunneled under the skin to the patient's opposite side.
  - A pocket for the attachment is made that will serve as the location of the future IPG. The location is the patient's opposite side below the iliac crest with sufficient subcutaneous fat to comfortably protect the device. A 3-cm skin incision is made and the tissue dissected to create a small pocket.
  - The tunneler device is inserted into the pocket approximately 2 cm beneath the skin and angled toward the lead. The device is gently advanced through the fat and the tip fed out through the lead skin incision. This tunnel should remain deep to the skin to decrease the risk of future exposure.
  - The tip of the tunneler is then unscrewed and removed. The metal tunneler is removed from its sheath. The lead is gently fed into the tunneler sheath as deep as possible until the lead tip is seen at the opposite end, inside the tube, exiting the previously made pocket. The tunneler and lead are grasped and pulled through the pocket side such that the tunneler is removed and the lead lays flat inside the tunnel.
- The extension wire is then attached.
  - A small plastic "boot" is slid onto the lead and the lead is fed into the extension wire which also has a small boot. The enclosed screwdriver is used to tighten the connections. The screwdriver should be turned and two small "clicks" heard. Care should be taken not to bend the connection or over-tighten.
  - The boots are then slid over the connection to ensure a water-tight seal. Two absorbable sutures are then affixed to either side of the boots to help prevent dislodging and leakage of fluid into the boots.
- The extension wire is then tunneled under the skin.
  - A small skin puncture is made at a location distant from the pocket. The tunneler is inserted into the puncture site and advanced, again deep to the skin, toward the pocket until it exits the skin. The tip and metal portion are removed and the extension lead fed through the tunneler, and slide out the puncture site as previously performed. This should result in the boot-covered extension connection being gently laid inside the pocket and the extension wire exiting the skin through the puncture site.
- The incisions are then closed.
  - The pocket is then copiously irrigated and hemostasis achieved. This step is critical to prevent hematoma and wound separation postoperatively. The subcuticular tissue is closed with absorbable sutures and the skin closed with sutures or skin staples. The two additional skin puncture incisions are similarly irrigated and closed.
- The extension lead is attached to the external power box.

- All incisions can be covered with bandages or Steri-Strips (3M, St. Paul, MN). Many describe additional coverage to help prevent inadvertent dislodging, pain, or infection. For example, with folded 4- × 4-gauze sponges covered with Tegaderm (3M, St. Paul, MN) horizontally across the patient's lower back covering the pocket incision, the small midline incisions, and the exposed extension wire until the anterior border of the iliac crest.
- In the recovery area, the patient is instructed on device management, programming, symptom records, and troubleshooting. The patient should follow-up with the surgeon to review results of the trial. Trial durations range from 1 to 4 weeks and depend on outcomes, surgeon and patient preference, and infection risk (see **Pearls and Pitfalls**).

Staged Implantation: Second Stage

- The patient is positioned and draped as in the first stage with the exception of level of anesthesia. The patient does not need to respond or interact with the surgeon for the second stage and can therefore receive more sedation if desired.
- The extension wire is disconnected from the tined lead.
    - The pocket skin incision is opened sharply with care *not to incise the underlying lead*. Blunt dissection is used to open the pocket and identify the connection which can be gently lifted out of the incision.
    - The two sutures alongside the boots are removed and the boots slid along the wires to expose the connection. The screwdriver is then used to disconnect the extension lead in a reverse manner from that performed in the first stage. The extension lead is then passed off of the field.
- The IPG is then attached.
    - The IPG is connected to the tined lead in a similar manner to that described for the temporary extension lead.
- The IPG is then placed inside the pocket. If necessary, blunt dissection can be used to enlarge the pocket to ensure sufficient space to accommodate the IPG with the wires beneath. This to protect the wires from infection, pain, or dislodging.
- Hemostasis is achieved and the pocket closed and dressed as described previously for the first stage.
- In the recovery area the patient is instructed on device management, programming, symptom records, and troubleshooting. The patient should follow-up with the surgeon for postoperative wound check in 4 to 6 weeks.

Percutaneous Evaluation

- This approach is most often used when the first stage is performed in the office setting, with or without fluoroscopy.
- The patient is positioned and draped in a similar manner as described above as is the procedure for identification of landmarks and foramen needle insertion. The exception is the placement of the PNE lead instead of the tined lead.
- Following insertion and confirmation of proper location of the PNE lead, the wire does not need to be tunneled as performed with the tined lead.
- The puncture incision and lead are covered with bandages and the PNE wire is attached to the external power supply.

Sacral Neuromodulation: Special Considerations

Assessment of Test Phase Results

- After stage one of either the staged implantation or PNE the results are reviewed with the patient. The criteria for success are detailed above.
- If the patient has undergone staged implantation, the extension lead is disconnected at this office visit to minimize infection risk.
  - The bandages are removed. The extension wire is placed on gentle traction and cut as close to the skin as possible such that the end of the wire retracts beneath the skin. The site is then covered with a small bandage.
  - The patient is instructed that her symptoms will likely return to baseline, as the device has been disconnected.
- If the patient has undergone PNE, the wire is removed at this office visit. Gentle traction will slide the wire out of the incision which can then be covered with a small bandage.

Wound Infection

- Incision cellulitis often resolves with a course of oral antibiotics.
- Cases of persistent infection or abscess often require removal of all device parts.
- Patients with a history of wound infection requiring explanation are candidates for repeat insertion, typically after significant time is allowed for infection resolution (approximately 3 months). In such cases, a combined approach can be used wherein the permanent tined lead and IPG are inserted in one stage as the patient has presumably demonstrated treatment benefit previously and does not require a repeat test phase.

PEARLS AND PITFALLS

BLADDER LANDMARKS

- Apply gentle traction on an inflated Foley catheter to bring the balloon to a comfortable position in the bladder neck. Palpation on the vaginal side will identify the location of the bladder neck. Measurement from the bladder neck to urethral meatus and identification of the midpoint reveal the mid-urethra which can be marked for assistance with incision planning.

CREATION OF VAGINAL INCISION

- Care should be used when handling vaginal epithelial edges. Rough tissue handling, prolonged use of Allis or tissue clamps, or macerating the edge during tunnel creation can devitalize the vaginal epithelium. This can result in poor tissue healing and may cause subsequent mesh exposure.

PERIURETHRAL DISSECTION

- When creating the tunnels for mid-urethral sling (MUS) placement, care should be taken not to penetrate the periurethral fascia.

CYSTOSCOPY

- Diagnostic cystoscopy is typically performed using a 17-French rigid cystoscope. Lens angle is 0 degree for visualization of the urethra and 30 or 70 degrees for visualization of the bladder neck, anterior bladder, ureters, or for thorough evaluation for trocar perforation at the time of sling procedures.

URINARY RETENTION

- Transient urinary retention may be frustrating to patients and physicians. Consider instructing patients on self-catheterization preoperatively to decrease anxiety and office visits postoperatively.

FLUOROSCOPY

- May be used for sacral neuromodulation. Requires physician licensure or registration in some states (https://www.aart.org).

SACRAL NEUROMODULATION TEST PHASE

- If insufficient results are achieved, the patient may be seen in the office for device reprogramming. The test phase can be extended to allow for evaluation of the results of the second reprogramming.

POSTOPERATIVE CARE

- Postoperative care following urogynecologic procedures is similar to that for other benign gynecologic surgery (see **Table 5.6**).
- Prophylactic antibiotics are **recommended** for the following procedures:
  - Vaginal surgery and sling placement: Guidelines from the surgical care improvement project (SCIP) recommend using a first- or second-generation cephalosporin for 24 hours.
  - Sacral neuromodulation: Manufacturer guidelines recommend antibiotic use in general to prevent implant infection.
- Continuous bladder drainage is **not required** for the following procedures:
  - Prolapse surgery and sling placement: Overall risk of urinary retention is low and does not justify continuous drainage in all patients. The decision should be made on a case-by-case basis and patients should be counseled on the risks and benefits of multiple options. Patients at high risk for postoperative retention may remain with an indwelling catheter or be instructed on self-catheterization to decrease anxiety and to avoid visits to emergency facilities.
- Continuous bladder drainage is **not recommended** for the following procedures:
  - Transurethral bulking, cystoscopic procedures, and procedures not involving the bladder or urethra: Following successful urination patients may be discharged home without drainage.
- Physical activity restriction is **recommended** for the following procedures:
  - Prolapse surgery, sling placement, vaginal surgery: Sexual activity and aerobic exercise should be limited in the immediate postoperative period.

Table 5.6 Summary of Recommendations Following Urogynecologic Surgery

Treatment	Recommendation
Antibiotics	• *Recommended:* vaginal surgery, sling procedures, neuromodulation
Bladder drainage	• *Not required:* vaginal surgery and sling procedures • *Not recommended:* cystoscopic procedures
Activity restrictions	• *Recommended:* vaginal surgery, sling procedures, neuromodulation • *Not recommended:* cystoscopic procedures

- Follow-up evaluation is **recommended** for the following procedures:
  - Approximately 2 weeks for patients at high risk of urinary retention following anti-incontinence procedures.
  - Approximately 4 to 6 weeks in low-risk patients following vaginal surgery and neuromodulation.

OUTCOMES

Stress Urinary Incontinence

- **Mid-urethral slings**
  - Approximately 84% (range 76% to 89%) of patients report being cured or dry after synthetic MUSs at 48 months or longer.[1]
- **Pubovaginal slings**
  - Approximately 82% (range 67% to 93%) of patients report being cured or dry after autologous pubovaginal slings at 4 years or longer.[1]
- **Transurethral bulking**
  - Approximately 30% (range 18% to 45%) of patients are cured or dry at 48 months while 66% are improved.[1] The procedure can be repeated if needed.

Urinary Urge Incontinence

- **Cystoscopic injection of botulinum toxin**
  - Average decrease in urinary frequency is four episodes per day, and decrease in UI episodes is three per day. Duration of action ranges from 3 to 12 months and up to 66% of patients experience resolution of UI. The procedure can be repeated if needed.
- **Sacral neuromodulation**
  - Overall success is approximately 76% to 86%, with improvement in urinary frequency, nocturia, UI episodes, and quality of life.[8] Duration of action depends on frequency of use and battery life. Batteries can be surgically replaced. Improvement in quality of life has been demonstrated related to improvement in urinary, fecal, and sexual function.

COMPLICATIONS

- **Mid-urethral slings**
  - Most common perioperative complications include urinary tract infection, urinary retention, and voiding dysfunction, which are reported in approximately 3% to 5% of patients and increase with time.
  - Mesh-related complications such as vaginal exposure, visceral erosion, and pelvic pain.
- **Pubovaginal slings**
  - Most common side effects are similar to those described for MUSs but with slightly higher rates of urinary retention and urinary urgency.

- **Transurethral bulking**
  - Most common side effects are similar to those described for MUSs but with lower rates of occurrence. More commonly transient urinary discomfort is seen.
- **Cystoscopic injection of botulinum toxin**
  - Most commonly reported side effects include urinary tract infections in 13% to 44% and urinary retention in 9% to 25% depending on medication dosage.
- **Sacral neuromodulation**
  - Most commonly reported adverse events include an uncomfortable sensation of stimulation or implant site pain in 8% to 10%, and lead migration or implant site infection or repeat surgery in 3%.

KEY REFERENCES

1. Dmochowski RR, Blaivas JM, Gormley EA, et al; Female Stress Urinary Incontinence Update Panel of the American Urological Association Education and Research, Inc. Update of AUA guideline on the surgical management of female stress urinary incontinence. *J Urol.* 2010;183(5):1906–1914.
2. Madhuvrata P, Cody JD, Ellis G, Herbison GP, Hay-Smith EJ. Which anticholinergic drug for overactive bladder symptoms in adults. *Cochrane Database Syst Rev.* 2012;1:CD005429.
3. Gormley EA, Lightner DJ, Faraday M, Vasavada SP; American Urological Association; Society of Urodynamics, Female Pelvic Medicine. Diagnosis and treatment of overactive bladder (non-neurogenic) in adults: AUA/SUFU guideline amendment. *J Urol.* 2015;193(5):1572–1580.
4. Nager CW, Brubaker L, Litman HJ, et al; Urinary Incontinence Treatment Network. A randomized trial of urodynamic testing before stress-incontinence surgery. *N Engl J Med.* 2012;366(21):1987–1997.
5. Bakali E, Buckley BS, Hilton P, Tincello DG. Treatment of recurrent stress urinary incontinence after failed minimally invasive synthetic suburethral tape surgery in women. *Cochrane Database Syst Rev.* 2013;(2):CD009407.
6. Rehman H, Bezerra CC, Bruschini H, Cody JD. Traditional suburethral sling operations for urinary incontinence in women. *Cochrane Database Syst Rev.* 2011;(1):CD001754.
7. Kirchin V, Page T, Keegan PE, Atiemo K, Cody JD, McClinton S. Urethral injection therapy for urinary incontinence in women. *Cochrane Database Syst Rev.* 2012;(2):CD003881.
8. Noblett K, Siegel S, Mangel J, et al. Results of a prospective, multicenter study evaluating quality of life, safety, and efficacy of sacral neuromodulation at twelve months in subjects with symptoms of overactive bladder. *Neurourol Urodyn.* 2016;35(2):246–251.
9. Duthie JB, Vincent M, Herbison GP, Wilson DI, Wilson D. Botulinum toxin injections for adults with overactive bladder syndrome. *Cochrane Database Syst Rev.* 2011;(12):CD005493.
10. Committee Opinion No. 604: OnabotulinumtoxinA and the bladder. *Obstet Gynecol.* 2014;123(6):1408–1411.
11. Ulmsten U, Henriksson L, Johnson P, Varhos G. An ambulatory surgical procedure under local anesthesia for treatment of female urinary incontinence. *Int Urogynecol J Pelvic Floor Dysfunct.* 1996;7(2):81–85.

Chapter 6
Genitourinary Fistula

Erin M. Mellano, Lisa Rogo-Gupta

GENERAL PRINCIPLES
IMAGING AND OTHER DIAGNOSTICS
PREOPERATIVE PLANNING
SURGICAL MANAGEMENT
PROCEDURES AND TECHNIQUES
   Vaginal Approach for Vesicovaginal Fistulas
   Urethrovaginal Fistulas
   Abdominal Approach for Vesicovaginal Fistulas
   Laparoscopic and Robotic-Assisted Laparoscopic Techniques
PEARLS AND PITFALLS
POSTOPERATIVE CARE
OUTCOMES
COMPLICATIONS

Genitourinary Fistula

Erin M. Mellano, Lisa Rogo-Gupta

GENERAL PRINCIPLES

Definition

- A genitourinary (GU) fistula is an abnormal connection between the genital and urinary tract. This connection can involve the bladder (vesicovaginal), uterus (vesicouterine), ureter (ureterovaginal), or urethra (urethrovaginal) (Fig. 6.1).
- Obstetric GU fistulas have virtually been eliminated from industrialized nations, but continue to dominate as the primary etiology in the developing world. They result from obstructed labor; during which time the soft tissues in the maternal pelvis become trapped between the fetal head and the bony pelvis. This entrapment leads to ischemic necrosis of the walls between the vagina and surrounding structures and the resulting damage leaves women with a defect connecting the genital and urinary tracts (Fig. 6.2).
  - GU fistulas represent a significant maternal morbidity. Women are often abandoned by their husbands and are unable to serve a functional role in their community due to their continuous incontinence.
- In developed countries, GU fistulas are rare. When they occur, they are often a result of unrecognized urinary tract injury during pelvic surgery. Other etiologies include pelvic radiation, cancer, trauma, and congenital anomalies.

Physical Examination

- General pelvic examination: Please see Table 5.1.
- Telltale signs of a GU fistula on physical exam include:
  - Pooling of urine in the vaginal vault
  - Dimpling or scar in the vagina
  - Granulation tissue overlying the fistulous tract in the vagina
  - Urine dermatitis (Fig. 6.3)
  - Sequelae of obstructed labor: vaginal stenosis and contracture, amenorrhea, symphyseal separation, and foot drop

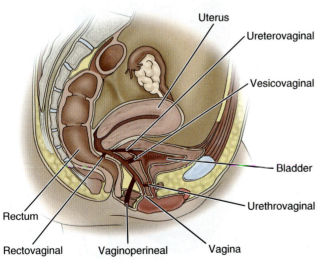

Figure 6.1. Illustration depicts three different types of genitourinary fistulas: vesicovaginal fistula, uterovaginal fistula, and urethrovaginal fistula. (From Farrell M. *Smeltzer & Bares Textbook of Medical-Surgical Nursing.* 4th ed. Philadelphia, PA: Wolters Kluwer; 2016.)

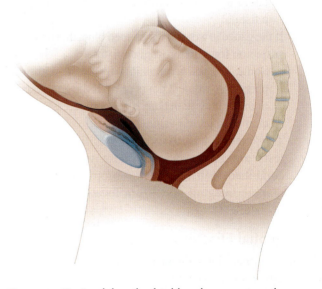

Figure 6.2. During labor the fetal head compresses the tissues between the bladder and the vagina. When labor is prolonged, blood flow to the compressed tissue is blocked, and the tissues undergo necrosis secondary to the decrease in blood flow.

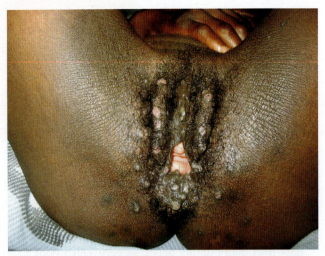

Figure 6.3. Vulvar urine dermatitis.

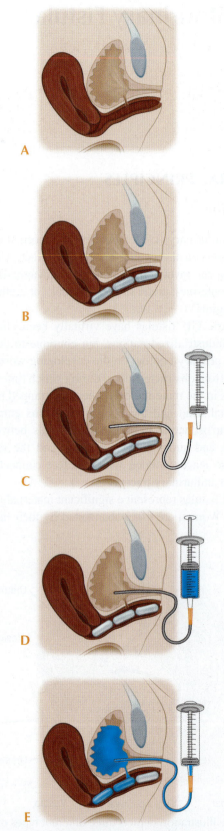

Figure 6.4. Series of illustrations depicting the "tampon test." A: Sagittal view of the pelvis with a vesicovaginal fistula. B: Gauze placed in the vagina. C: Catheter placed into the bladder with a syringe next to the pelvis. D: Blue-dyed fluid instilled into the bladder. E: Fluid leaking out of the bladder through the fistula onto the gauze in the vagina.

- If the source of the urinary incontinence cannot be readily determined, bladder instillation with blue dye can aid in diagnosis. This technique, along with vaginal packing is frequently referred to as the "tampon test." It is performed as follows (Fig. 6.4):
  - Place gauze in the vagina.
  - Retrograde fill of the bladder with blue-stained fluid.
  - After several minutes, remove the gauze.
  - If the gauze is stained blue, this increases suspicion for a fistula.
    - If only the distal aspect of the gauze is blue, this could be from urethral incontinence, rather than a fistula.
  - If the gauze is wet and not stained blue, this increases suspicion for a ureterovaginal fistula.
    - Some suggest combining this test with oral phenazopyridine 2 hours prior. If the gauze stains orange rather than blue, it further increases suspicion for a ureterovaginal fistula.
  - The overall sensitivity and specificity of these tests are unknown, and these tests are often combined with cystourethroscopy and/or radiographic imaging to confirm location and course of fistula.

Differential Diagnosis

- Stress urinary incontinence
- Overflow incontinence
- Ectopic ureter
- Peritoneal vaginal fistula
  - Intraperitoneal fluid collection with vaginal cuff dehiscence
- Vaginal discharge from infection, abscess, or fluid collection

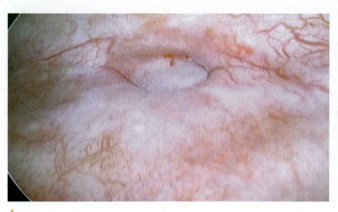 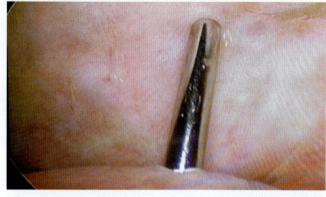

Figure 6.5. Post-hysterectomy fistula. **A:** Cystoscopic view of vesicovaginal fistula after laparoscopic hysterectomy. **B:** Probe is placed through the fistula tract.

Nonoperative Management

- For vesicovaginal fistulas if the diagnosis is made immediately (within 7 days), conservative treatment with continuous bladder drainage should be attempted as a first-line treatment.
  - An exception to this recommendation is for instances of fistulas secondary to radiation. These fistulas often have a delayed presentation, and are unlikely to heal from continuous bladder drainage alone.
  - Approximately 15% to 20% of small fistulas close spontaneously with continuous bladder drainage.
  - Positive predictors of successful closure with conservative management include:
    - Fistulas <1 cm *if* the catheter is placed shortly after diagnosis
    - Early recognition and placement of catheter
  - There is no consensus on optimal drainage duration, but generally, the catheter is left in for 2 to 8 weeks.
- For ureterovaginal fistulas, ureteral stent placement should be used as a first-line treatment.
  - Cases that are amenable to ureteral stenting include those with:
    - Unilateral ureteral injury
    - Absence of kidney infection
    - Ureteral continuity
    - Reliable follow-up
- Stenting for 6 to 8 weeks is recommended, and results in closure in 60% to 70% of cases.

IMAGING AND OTHER DIAGNOSTICS

- If the fistula is readily identified on physical exam, additional imaging is not necessary for diagnosis, but may aid in surgical planning.

- **Cystourethroscopy** (Fig. 6.5A,B)
  - Cystourethroscopy is an excellent method for identifying fistulas and is useful for visualizing the location of the fistula communication in relation to the ureters. It can be helpful in complex fistula where the tract is oblique and/or the vesical injury is cribriform.
- **Voiding cystourethrography (VCUG)** (Figs. 6.6 and 6.7)
  - This is the first-line imaging technique for vesicovaginal, vesicouterine, and urethrovaginal fistulas.
- **Computed tomography (CT) urogram**
  - This is the preferred imaging technique to identify ureterovaginal fistulas.
- **Hysterogram/saline sonohysterogram**
  - This technique can help identify a connection if suspected between the abdominal cavity and the uterus.

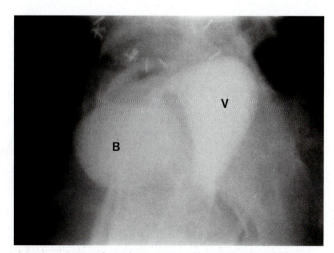

Figure 6.6. Lateral voiding cystourethrogram showing a vesicovaginal fistula. B = bladder; V = vagina. (From Dunnick R, Sandler C, Newhouse J. *Textbook of Uroradiology*. 5th ed. Philadelphia, PA: Wolters Kluwer; 2012.)

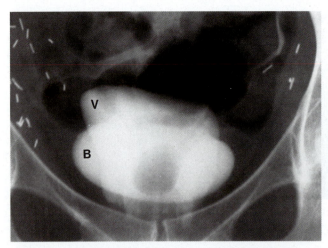

Figure 6.7. Anterior–posterior cystourethrogram showing vesicovaginal fistula. B = bladder; V = vagina. (From Dunnick R, Sandler C, Newhouse J. *Textbook of Uroradiology*. Philadelphia, PA: Wolters Kluwer; 2012.)

PREOPERATIVE PLANNING

- Identification of fistulous tract is critical.
- Timing of repair.
  - By convention, if a fistula is recognized within 72 hours, an immediate repair can be attempted. For fistulas presenting more than a few days after injury, specifically in the case of obstetric fistulas, repair is frequently delayed for several months to allow for resolution of inflammation.
  - For postsurgical fistulas, depending on characteristics of the fistula and tissue quality, a repair within the first 3 months is feasible.
  - For women with an active infection, repair should be delayed until the infection resolves.
- In instances in which a foreign body has caused the fistula, the foreign body, such as mesh, pessary, or permanent suture, must be removed before attempting to close the fistula.
- For vesicouterine or vesicocervical fistulas, if the fistula is recognized in the early postpartum period, it is recommended to wait at least 3 months, after uterine involution, to repair the defect.

SURGICAL MANAGEMENT

- A consensus on the ideal approach for surgical correction of GU fistula is lacking. The most important principle in GU fistula repair is to provide a tension-free, watertight closure, and the surgical route chosen should be the one that optimizes closure on first attempt. A transvaginal route is preferable for fistulas that can be accessed vaginally (urethrovaginal and most vesicovaginal fistulas); while a transabdominal route is preferred for high vesicovaginal without vaginal descent, some uterovaginal, and ureterovaginal fistulas.

Positioning

- GU fistula repairs are performed with the patient in the dorsal lithotomy position, similar to most other gynecologic procedures. Even in instances where the repair will be approached abdominally, access to the perineum is essential.
- Various lithotomy stirrups are available to assure patient safety and comfort, minimizing risk for related perioperative neuropathic injury (Fig. 6.8).

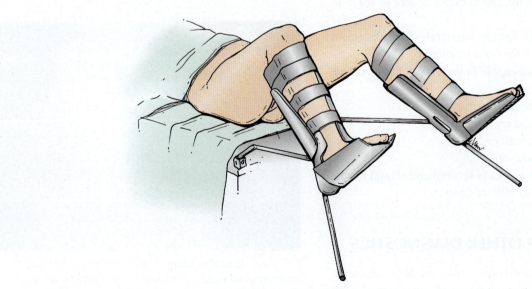

Figure 6.8. Lithotomy position. (From Jones HW, Rock JA. *Te Linde's Operative Gynecology*. 11th ed. Philadelphia, PA: Wolters Kluwer; 2015.)

- For laparoscopic procedures:
  - Patients should be placed in dorsal lithotomy position to allow adequate perineal access during the case.
  - The arms can be tucked to facilitate surgery.
  - It may be beneficial to place an additional intravenous line to ensure adequate access during the case.

Approach

- The vaginal approach is an appropriate approach for most GU fistulas. In a prospective cohort study of more than 1,200 women undergoing obstetric fistula repair, 95% of the fistulas were repaired vaginally.
- Vaginal approach
  - Vesicovaginal fistula
  - Urethrovaginal fistula
  - Vesicocervical fistula
- Abdominal approach is also acceptable and may be preferable in instances of:
  - Extensive scarring or tissue loss
  - Genital infibulation
  - Ureteric involvement
  - Vesicouterine fistulas
  - Concomitant abdominal pathology
- Ureterovaginal fistula
  - For ureterovaginal fistula the transabdominal route is preferred. This allows for ureteral dissection, reconstruction, or reimplantation when necessary.
  - This can be done via laparotomy or laparoscopy.

Vaginal Approach for Vesicovaginal Fistulas (Video 6.1)

- This procedure may be done under regional or general anesthesia.
- Adequate exposure of the fistula is imperative. If a narrow introitus limits visualization, an episiotomy-style incision or resection of intravaginal scar tissue can be performed to help facilitate access.
- A self-retaining vaginal retractor (such as Scott retractor) is vital to optimize visualization (Tech Fig. 6.1).
- If cystoscopy was not performed preoperatively, it can be done so in the operating room to determine the relationship of the fistula to the ureters. If the fistula is in close proximity to the ureter, a ureteral catheter or stent should be passed to facilitate identification of the ureter during the repair.

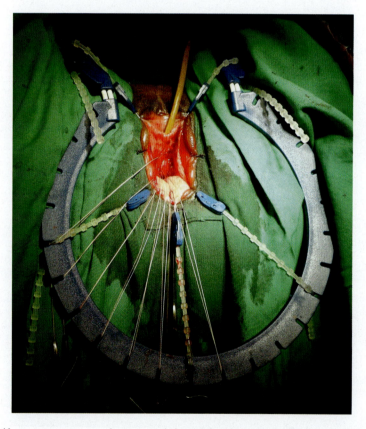

Tech Figure 6.1. Self-retaining retractor being used during fistula surgery. This retractor helps with visualization and with organization of sutures.

- A Foley catheter is placed in the urethra, and a blue dye test repeated in the operating room to map the area(s) of fistulas (see Tech Fig. 6.2; Video 6.2).
- A probe or a pediatric Foley catheter may be placed into the fistula to identify the tract and to demarcate the boundaries. If a pediatric catheter is used, it provides the added benefit of allowing traction to be placed on the fistula and to bring the fistula closer to the introitus (Tech Fig. 6.3).

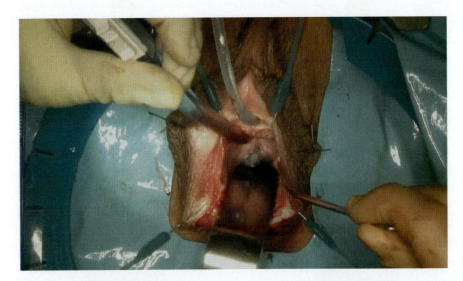

Tech Figure 6.2. After retrograde fill of bladder, blue dye is visualized from the bladder and out the fistula site in the vagina. This technique is often performed in the office and can be repeated in the operating room to identify the fistulous tract.

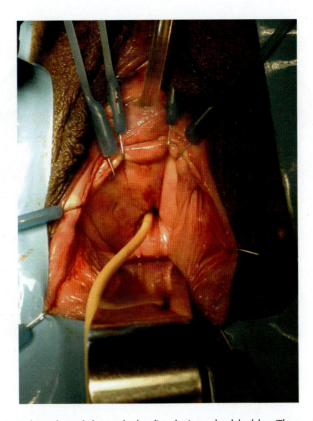

Tech Figure 6.3. Pediatric Foley placed through the fistula into the bladder. The pediatric Foley not only identifies the fistula opening and tract, but traction can be placed on the Foley to bring the fistula closer to the vaginal opening.

- Marking sutures of 3.0 delayed absorbable suture can be placed at the lateral aspects of the fistulous tract to demarcate the extent of the fistula.
- The fistula is circumscribed. The fistula tract does not have to be excised unless the edges appear necrotic or inflamed (Tech Fig. 6.4).

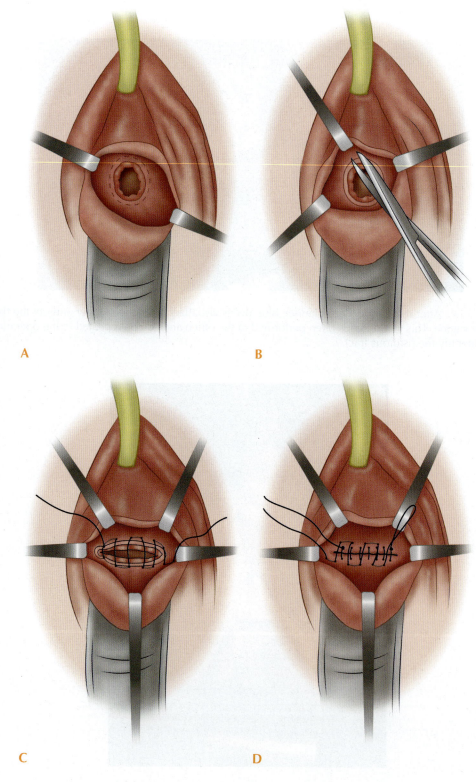

A   B

C   D

Tech Figure 6.4. Vesicovaginal fistula repair. A: The fistula. B: The vaginal epithelium is widely mobilized and dissected off of the underlying bladder. C: Interrupted sutures closing the fistula. D: A second layer of suture to reinforce the first layer.

- Vaginal tissue flaps are mobilized off of the underlying fibromuscular tissue using Metzenbaum scissors. Ample lateral dissection of the bladder from the full-thickness epithelium is important to ensure a tension-free repair.
- The bladder mucosa is closed with interrupted 2.0 or 3.0 delayed absorbable suture. For the first layer these sutures are placed and held until all sutures have been placed. They are then serially tied.
  - Integrity of the repair is assessed with a retrograde fill of the bladder with methylene blue–stained fluid.
  - The first layer should be watertight before proceeding.
  - The repair should be tension free.
- Closure is reinforced with at least a second layer of fibromuscular tissue of the bladder.
- If the tissue appears devitalized or densely scarred, a vascular pedicle should be harvested and interposed between the fibromuscular layer and the vaginal epithelium (see section on Tissue Interposition: Martius flap or peritoneal flap).
- The previously mobilized vaginal tissue flap is then closed, taking care to avoid overlapping suture lines.

Urethrovaginal Fistulas

- The approach and surgical steps are similar to that of a vaginal closure of a vesicovaginal fistula.
- If the defect is small, a primary repair over the Foley catheter can be performed (Tech Fig. 6.5).
  - Analogous to the vesicovaginal fistulas, the vaginal epithelium around the fistula is incised.
  - Vaginal tissue flaps are created. This can be done with either a cruciate incision or with an inverted-U incision.
  - The urethral mucosa is closed using 3.0 delayed absorbable suture over the Foley catheter. Ensure that with each suture placed, the catheter has not been incorporated into the repair.
  - Integrity should be assessed by backfilling the bladder with blue dye–stained solution.
  - The fibromuscular layer is used to reinforce the repair as a second layer.
  - If the tissue appears weak or compromised, a Martius flap can be used to reinforce the closure.
  - The vaginal epithelial skin flaps are then closed.

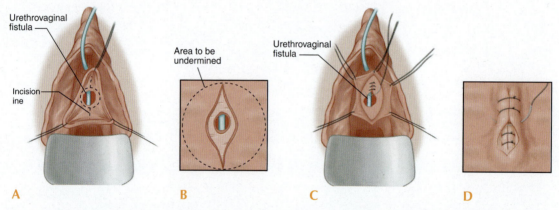

Tech Figure 6.5. Urethrovaginal fistula closure. **A:** Urethrovaginal fistula. **B:** Dissection of the vaginal epithelium off of the urethra. **C:** Closure of the urethra with interrupted sutures with the Foley catheter in place. **D:** Second reinforcing layer of suture.

Abdominal Approach for Vesicovaginal Fistulas

- The transabdominal route is preferred for fistulas that are not accessible from the vaginal route, or in instances of complex fistulas, in which ureteral reimplantation may be necessary.

Open Techniques

- Open O'Conor transperitoneal supravesical technique is the traditional abdominal closure method.
- The patient should be placed in the dorsal lithotomy position (see **Fig. 6.8**).
- The abdomen and the perineum should be sterilely prepped and a Foley catheter is placed into the bladder.
- A low vertical midline incision or a low transverse incision is an acceptable option, depending on the anticipated findings and previous scars (**Tech Fig. 6.6**).

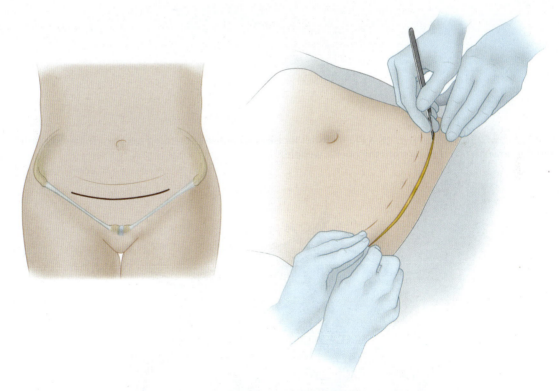

Tech Figure 6.6. This image depicts the location of a Pfannenstiel incision.

- This technique can be performed either intra- or extraperitoneally. If the peritoneum is entered, the bowel should be packed away and a self-retaining retractor utilized (Tech Fig. 6.7).
- The space of Retzius is accessed and the bladder is bisected along the sagittal plane, starting anteriorly, until the fistulous tract is reached. If the ureters are close to the fistula, stents should be passed (Tech Fig. 6.8).

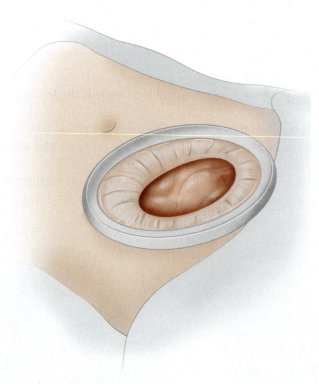

Tech Figure 6.7. This image depicts a Pfannenstiel incision with a self-retaining retractor in the incision and the bowel packed away from the operative field.

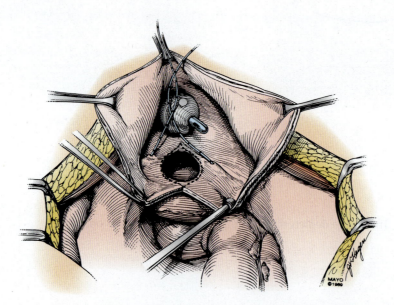

Tech Figure 6.8. The dome of the bladder is opened to visualize the fistula. Ureteral stents can be placed. The bladder is incised up to the level site of the fistula. (From Lee RA. *Atlas of Gynecologic Surgery*. Philadelphia, PA: WB Saunders; 1992. Used with permission of Mayo Foundation for Medical Education and Research. All rights reserved.)

- The bladder and vagina are separated and the fistulous tract is excised (Tech Fig. 6.9).
- The vagina and bladder are each closed with 2.0 or 3.0 delayed absorbable sutures, and a vascular flap, usually of omentum, is interposed between the vagina and the bladder (Tech Figs. 6.10 to 6.12). The bladder is then closed in two layers.

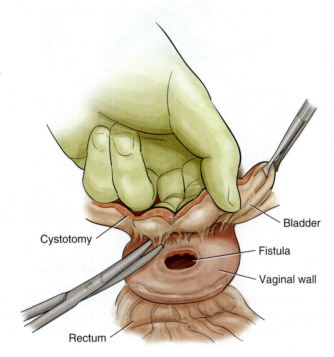

Tech Figure 6.9. The bladder and the vagina are separated and the fistulous tract can be excised. (From Lee RA. *Atlas of Gynecologic Surgery*. Philadelphia, PA: WB Saunders; 1992. Used with permission of Mayo Foundation for Medical Education and Research. All rights reserved.)

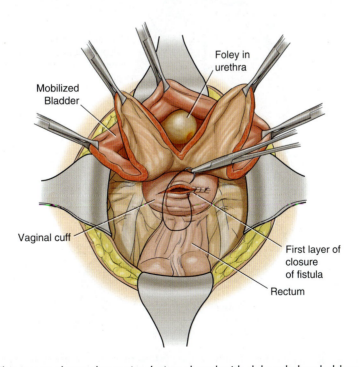

Tech Figure 6.10. This image shows the vagina being closed with delayed absorbable suture in a continuous fashion. (From Lee RA. *Atlas of Gynecologic Surgery*. Philadelphia, PA: WB Saunders; 1992. Used with permission of Mayo Foundation for Medical Education and Research. All rights reserved.)

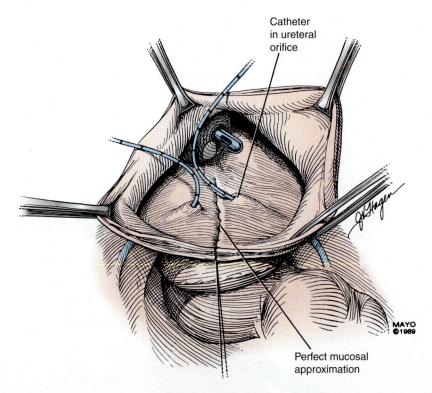

Tech Figure 6.11. This image depicts the closure of the fistula on the bladder side. The bladder fistula is closed in two layers with interrupted delayed absorbable suture. (From Lee RA. *Atlas of Gynecologic Surgery*. Philadelphia, PA: WB Saunders; 1992. Used with permission of Mayo Foundation for Medical Education and Research. All rights reserved.)

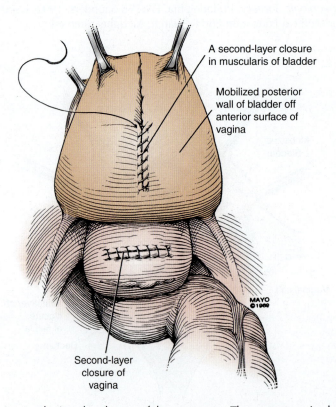

Tech Figure 6.12. This image depicts the closure of the cystotomy. The cystotomy is closed in two layers with running delayed absorbable suture. Interposition of a tissue flap can be placed between the bladder and the vagina. (From Lee RA. *Atlas of Gynecologic Surgery*. Philadelphia, PA: WB Saunders; 1992. Used with permission of Mayo Foundation for Medical Education and Research. All rights reserved.)

- Many modifications to this technique have been made. The basic principle remains, with a transvesical incision to access the fistula.
  - Advantages of this technique include high closure rate, wide mobilization, removal of scar tissue, and tension-free closure, and it allows for ureteral reimplantation if necessary. Despite some of the noted advantages, the associated morbidity of extensive bladder bisection has prompted surgeons to develop modifications to this technique.
- **Extravesical approaches** with minimal dissection of the bladder have been described with similar success rates to the traditional O'Conor technique and overall have decreased associated morbidity.
  - This technique avoids bivalving the bladder.
  - The fistulous tract can be demarcated with a stent in the fistula.
  - The vesicovaginal reflection is identified. If not readily seen, the bladder can be retrograde filled to better demarcate the borders.
  - A vaginal stent or end-to-end anastomosis (EEA) sizer can be placed in the vagina to provide a firm surface for dissection.
  - Sharp dissection is carried down to the fistulous tract.
  - The tract is excised.
  - Distal dissection past the fistula is continued an additional centimeter or two, to completely separate the bladder and the vagina.
  - The bladder side is repaired with 2.0 or 3.0 delayed absorbable suture in two layers. The integrity of the repair should be checked after the first layer is closed with a retrograde fill of the bladder using methylene blue–stained solution.
  - Cystoscopy should be performed to confirm bilateral ureteral function.
  - The vagina is closed using 2.0 delayed absorbable suture.
  - A vascular flap should be interposed between the two tissue planes, in most cases.

Laparoscopic and Robotic-Assisted Laparoscopic Techniques

- Laparoscopic techniques for transabdominal repair of fistulas are an attractive minimally invasive option, decreasing morbidity associated with exploratory surgery. These have been described utilizing trans- or extravesical approaches. Due to the frequent need to perform extensive suturing deep in the pelvis, robotic-assisted laparoscopy may provide additional advantages, with increased visualization and ease of suturing, over traditional laparoscopy.

Vesicouterine or Vesicocervical Fistulas

- These fistulas tend to be repaired transabdominally, via either an open or laparoscopic approach.
- If vaginal access and repair of a vesicocervical fistula are feasible, this route is also acceptable.
- The patient is prepared in the same way as previously described for open or laparoscopic technique.
- Either a transperitoneal or a transvesical approach is acceptable.
- It is not necessary to perform a concomitant hysterectomy.
- Once adequate exposure has been obtained, the bladder is carefully dissected away from the uterus, and the dissection is carried down caudal to the fistulous tract.
- The dissection of the bladder off the cervix of the uterus is often more tedious and tenuous than simple vesicovaginal fistula.
- Attention to the caudal margin of the bladder injury should be prioritized as this is often the most difficult to secure.
- The bladder is then repaired with 2.0 or 3.0 delayed absorbable suture in two layers.
- The uterine defect is repaired and a vascular tissue flap of omentum or peritoneum should be used to separate the two repairs.

Vascular Tissue Interposition

- While many fistulas are amenable to repair with simple, tension-free, multilayer closure, there are some fistulas in which the interposition of well-vascularized tissue is essential.
- Vascular tissue interposition flaps should be used in fistula repair that are:
  - More complex
  - Occur secondary to cancer or radiation
  - Previous repair failures
  - Devitalized tissue
- For transvaginal approach, interposition options include:
  - Martius fat pad
  - Peritoneal flap
- Abdominal approach flaps include:
  - Omentum
  - Peritoneum
  - Rectus abdominus muscle

Martius Fat Pad Graft

- This is an easily accessible source of vascularized tissue for distal to mid-vaginal fistulas (urethrovaginal, vesicovaginal, and rectovaginal) that are repaired transvaginally. Blood supply to the Martius flap is derived from the external pudendal artery superiorly and from the internal pudendal artery inferiorly. Lateral blood supply is derived from the obturator artery (Tech Fig. 6.13).
- The patient must have adequate labial fat for this to be a possible procedure.
- The primary closure of the urethrovaginal or vesicovaginal fistula is as described above with traditional fistula repair until the point of closing the vaginal epithelium.

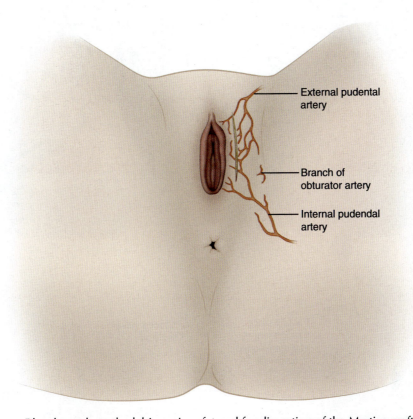

Tech Figure 6.13. Blood supply to the labia majora fat pad for dissection of the Martius graft.

- The Martius graft is harvested from the right or left labia majora. Choice of side should depend on the patient's anatomy and fistula location (Tech Fig. 6.14).
- A 6- to 8-cm incision is made in the labia majora and sharp dissection is used to mobilize the bulbocavernosus fat pad. Dissection is carried down to the fascia.
- Superiorly, the external pudendal artery is ligated and transected, leaving a broad fat pad base with intact blood supply from the branch of the internal pudendal artery.

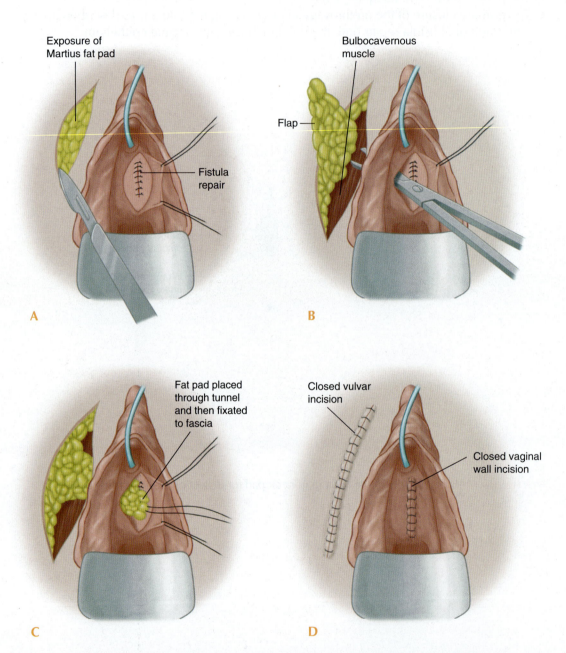

Tech Figure 6.14. This series of images depicts surgical approach to preparing and transferring the Martius fat pad graft. **A:** The first photo shows the incision made in the labia majora. **B:** The second photo shows the dissection and mobilization of the fat pad. Dissection is carried down to the fascia. Depending on the ease of mobilization and on the location of the fistula, either the ventral or the dorsal portion of the graft can be transferred. In this series of illustrations, the dorsal portion of the graft is transferred, and therefore, the internal pudendal artery is ligated and transected. The graft maintains its blood supply from the external pudendal artery. **C:** The third illustration shows the graft being transferred through a tunnel made in the vagina. The graft is passed through this tunnel and attached to sutures that were preplaced in the periurethral or perivesical tissue overlying the fistula closure. **D:** The last photo shows the closure of the vaginal epithelium over the graft.

- An incision is then made in the wall of the vagina to allow for transfer of the graft into the vagina. A tunnel is created to allow for passage of the graft to the fistula site.
- Stay sutures of 2.0 delayed absorbable material are placed around the periurethral tissue overlying the fistula and the Martius graft is attached to these sutures. The vaginal epithelium is then closed over the graft.
- The vulvar incision is irrigated and closed. The subcutaneous layer is closed with 2.0 delayed absorbable suture, and the epithelial layer is closed with 4.0 Monocryl in a running subcuticular fashion.

Transvaginal Peritoneal Flap
- For high vaginal-vault vesicovaginal fistulas, the peritoneum can be utilized as a vascular tissue layer to interpose between the fistula repair and the epithelium (Tech Fig. 6.15).
- The fistula should be repaired as above, with mobilization of vaginal epithelium, closure of bladder mucosa in first layer with a second layer of perivesical tissue.
- The peritoneum is mobilized in the cul-de-sac by sharp dissection and advanced over the repair.
- If the peritoneum is entered, it should be closed.
- The vaginal epithelium is then closed over the flap.

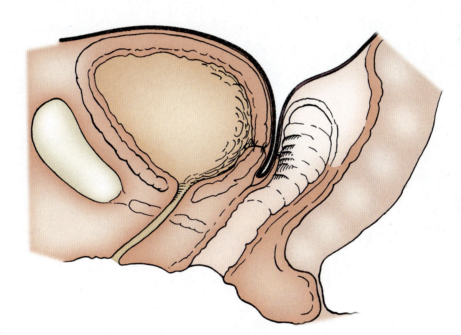

Tech Figure 6.15. Interposition of peritoneum between the vagina and the bladder. (Modified from Raz S, Bregg KJ, Nitti VW, Sussman E. Transvaginal repair of vesicovaginal fistula using a peritoneal flap. J Urol. 1993;150:56–59.)

Other Types of Vascular Flaps

Transvaginal Labial Flap
- These flaps are most useful in complex cases with loss of vaginal epithelium, precluding a primary vaginal closure. A full-thickness flap provides a vascular layer and tissue coverage.
- As described by Eilber et al. this flap is created by making a U-incision from the area of repair to the outer edge of the labia.
- The flap is rotated to cover the fistula.
- The vaginal epithelium is not covered over this flap.
- This flap is particularly useful when there is a paucity of vascularized vaginal epithelium.

Transvaginal Gluteal Flap
- This is a full-thickness pediculated flap that can provide vascularized tissue and tissue coverage, and should be considered in cases of vaginal stenosis, foreshortening, or extensive scarring.

Transabdominal Omental Flap
- When possible, the omentum is an ideal source for tissue interposition in fistula repair (Tech Fig. 6.16).

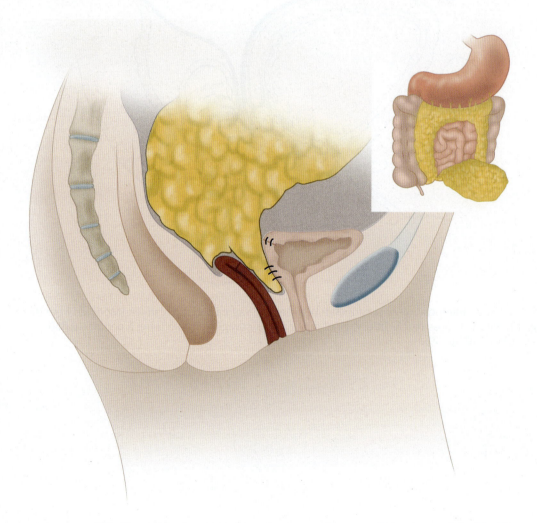

Tech Figure 6.16. This illustration shows omentum interposed between the vagina and the bladder.

- The omentum often needs to be mobilized to bring it to the pelvis.
  - Key points in mobilization:
    - Blood supply to the omentum must be preserved. It comes from the gastroepiploic arteries along the greater curvature of the stomach, and these must be carefully identified during mobilization.
    - Care must be taken to not have any traction on the omentum.
    - A vertical abdominal incision may facilitate omental mobilization easier than a low transverse incision.
  - Length of omentum needed to reach the pelvis in a tension-free manner should be determined prior to starting the dissection.
  - Mobilization can be initiated from the right at the hepatic flexure, or from the left at the greater curvature.
  - Care must be taken to ligate the vascular arcades. This can be done with suture ligation or with advanced electrocautery sealing devices.
  - Once the omentum is mobilized, it can be moved down to the pelvis to cover the repair site.

Transabdominal Peritoneal Flap
- Peritoneal flaps are especially useful in cases where an omental flap is not feasible.
- Peritoneum can be used from nearby peritoneum covering the bladder dome, lateral pelvic peritoneum, or anterior abdominal wall peritoneum.

PEARLS AND PITFALLS

CONSERVATIVE MANAGEMENT

○ Continuous bladder drainage with an indwelling catheter may result in closure of small, simple vesicovaginal fistulas (VVFs) in 10% to 20% of cases. Can be attempted to 6 to 12 weeks. For ureterovaginal fistulas, an attempt to pass a stent should be made and left in place for 6 to 8 weeks. In 60% to 70% of ureterovaginal fistula cases, the fistula will close with conservative management.

TIMING OF SURGERY

○ Surgery should be performed when the tissue is free of inflammation and induration. If the fistula is recognized within the first 72 hours of when it occurred, an immediate surgical repair is feasible. If an infection is present, one should wait until the infection has cleared before attempting surgical repair.

ROUTE OF SURGERY

○ Though vaginal approach is ideal for most fistulas, the best surgical route is the one in which the surgeon feels most confident in being able to adequately repair the fistula on the first attempt. The most important aspect of the fistula repair is to have a tension-free repair with a watertight seal.

USE OF A VASCULAR PEDICLE GRAFT

○ Vascular tissue grafts should be considered when the fistula is secondary to radiation; more complex; recurrent; or in devitalized tissue. Grafts that can be used include Martius labial fat pad grafts, full-thickness skin flap grafts, omentum, or peritoneum.

POSTOPERATIVE CARE

○ An indwelling catheter should be left in place for 2 to 3 weeks after the procedure. Fistula integrity should be assessed prior to removing the catheter.

POSTOPERATIVE CARE

- Routine instructions for postoperative care are similar to that for other benign gynecologic surgeries.

Antibiotics

- *Recommended:* Intraoperative prophylactic antibiotics have been shown to be beneficial in GU fistula repairs and are recommended with level I evidence.
- *Commonly used:* There is no consensus regarding the duration of postoperative prophylaxis.
  - There are limited data to suggest that postoperative antibiotics reduce the rate of bacteriuria, pyuria, febrile morbidity, and gram-negative isolates in patients' urine in surgical patients who undergo bladder drainage for at least 24 hours postoperatively.
- Daily postoperative prophylactic antibiotics should be considered for the duration of the indwelling urinary catheter.
- Antibiotic choice should cover gram-negative and gram-positive bacteria; however, no recommendation exists of type of antibiotic or of the dosing.

Anticholinergic Medication

- *Occasionally used:* Anticholinergic medications are sometimes given to help with troublesome bladder spasms.

Continuous Bladder Drainage

- *Recommended and required:* Postoperative continuous bladder drainage is imperative to successful fistula repair. Generally, the catheter is left in for 2 to 3 weeks. In a retrospective study comparing 10, 12, or 14 days of catheter drainage, there was no significant difference

in repair breakdown rate for any of the time points. We generally recommend a minimum of 14 days of continuous bladder drainage, and will increase this time period if it appears that the patient has healing complications.
- *Commonly used:* Suprapubic catheters can be used in conjunction with, or in lieu of transurethral catheters.
    - Patients may find these more comfortable and easier to manage than transurethral catheters.
    - In instances where additional bladder irrigation may be warranted, having two sources of bladder drainage may prove helpful.
    - A transurethral catheter should always be used in instances of urethrovaginal fistulas. Using a silastic Foley catheter is often more comfortable for prolonged drainage and the smooth, silicone exterior coating can reduce calcification buildup.
- Follow-up visit for assessment of repair integrity and to remove the catheter.
    - Vesicovaginal or urethrovaginal fistulas
        - *Recommended:* Repair integrity should be assessed prior to catheter removal.
        - *Commonly done:*
            - A retrograde dye test of the repair can be performed through the urethral catheter and is most facile.
            - A voiding cystourethrogram may also be performed.
            - With a suprapubic catheter in place, the urethral catheter can be removed and a suprapubic cystogram is performed.
    - Ureterovaginal fistulas
        - *Recommended:* Ureteral integrity should be assessed at 6 to 8 weeks after stent is placed.
        - *Commonly done:*
            - A CT urogram can be performed prior to removing the stent.

OUTCOMES

Transvaginal Fistula Repair
- When reporting closure rate, alone, the highest rate of successful closure is with the first surgery and ranges between 80% and 97%.

Open Transabdominal Vesicovaginal Fistula Repair
- Success rate of O'Conor open technique ranges between 65% and 100%.
- The wide range in success rates reflects the heterogeneity of complexity and prior closure attempts in published reports.

Laparoscopic and Robotic-Assisted Vesicovaginal Fistula Repair
- Similar success rates have been published in case series reports of traditional laparoscopic, single-port laparoscopic, and robotic-assisted laparoscopic fistula repairs, ranging between 86% and 100%.
- Both trans- and extravesical approaches have been utilized.
- With the adoption of laparoscopic procedures, we anticipate that use of this modality will continue to grow for fistula care.

COMPLICATIONS

Intraoperative Complications
- Bleeding
- Ureteral injury
    - Ureteral catheterization can help prevent inadvertent damage to the ureters during repair.
    - Cystourethroscopy with intravenous methylene blue or sodium fluorescein may be used to assess ureteral function if there is any question of ureter compromise.

Early Postoperative Complications
- Vaginal bleeding
- Bladder spasms
- Infections
- Catheter dysfunction
    - Careful attention must be paid to ensure continuous bladder drainage. If the catheter clogs and the bladder retains urine, the chance of repair breakdown dramatically increases.
    - Some physicians will leave both a suprapubic and a urethral catheter in place to ensure adequate drainage.
    - Teaching the patient or a nurse how to gently flush the catheter is a vital skill if the catheter becomes clogged during the postoperative period.

Delayed Complications
- Urethral incontinence
    - Postrepair urethral incontinence is a common problem after fistula closure particularly when urethral closure mechanism is near repair. Between 10% and 55% of women with successful closures of the fistulas suffer from urethral incontinence as a result of the traumatic birth injury that lead to the fistula.
    - Risk factors for post-fistula closure incontinence include absence of bladder neck and proximal urethral involvement of the fistula.

- Different methods for treatment of postrepair incontinence have been suggested including urethral bulking agents, urethropexy and suburethral slings using fascia, biologic graft materials, or synthetic mesh.
- To avoid the potential morbidity of fistula recurrence from the placement of a suburethral sling under a previously compromised urethra, some have suggested interposition of a flap of vascularized tissue or biologic graft to separate the previous repair from the sling.
- The optimal techniques for post-obstetric fistula repair incontinence should be determined on an individual basis. The integrity of the tissues is oftentimes scarred and devascularized. Unlike traditional urethra incontinence, these women suffer from nonfunctional or absent urethral closing mechanisms. Autologous proximal urethral slings may be better tolerated than those with synthetic material; however, randomized controlled trials and long-term follow-up data are lacking.

- Fistula recurrence
- Persistence of nonfunctional vagina
  - It is well recognized that successful fistula closure does not necessarily result in return to normal vaginal function.
  - Postoperative sexual function has not been extensively studied in these patients. In many patients suffering from obstetric fistulas, vaginal atresia from scarring and necrosis precludes preservation of vaginal length at the time of the fistula repair. Elkins reported a 50% gynatresia rate after correction of fistulas greater than 4 cm in size.
  - In developed countries, where fistulas tend to be small and apical and often recognized prior to extensive vaginal damage, the ability to preserve vaginal capacity is often achieved.
  - In a recent prospective study of sexual function assessed by validated questionnaires, in patients with GU fistulas in the United States, an improvement in most of the domains was noted after repair, with no significant difference in amount of improvement whether repair was performed transabdominally or transvaginally.

SUGGESTED READINGS

Bai SW, Huh EH, Jung DJ, et al. Urinary tract injuries during pelvic surgery: incidence rates and predisposing factors. *Int Urogynecol J Pelvic Floor Dysfunct.* 2006;17:360–364.

Bengtson AM, Kopp D, Tang JH, Chipungu E, Moyo M, Wilkinson J. Identifying patients with vesicovaginal fistula at high risk of urinary incontinence after surgery. *Obstet Gynecol.* 2016;128(5):945–953.

Chen SS, Yang SH, Yang JM, Huang WC. Transvaginal repair of ureterovaginal fistula by Latzko technique. *Int Urogynecol J Pelvic Floor Dysfunct.* 2013;18(11):1381–1383.

Eilber KS, Kavaler E, Rodriguez LV, Rosenblum N, Raz S. Ten-year experience with transvaginal vesicovaginal fistula repair using tissue interposition. *J Urol.* 2003;169:1033–1036.

Frajzngier V, Ruminjo J, Asiimwe F, et al. Factors influencing choice of surgical route of repair of genitourinary fistula, and the influence of route of repair on surgical outcomes: findings from a prospective cohort study. *BJOG.* 2012;119:1344–1353.

Goel A, Goel S. Re: Pshak et al: Is tissue interposition always necessary in transvaginal repair of benign, recurrent vesicovaginal fistulae? Urology (2013;82:707–712). *Urology.* 2014;83(1):257.

Hilton P. Urogenital fistula in the UK: a personal case series managed over 25 years. *BJU Int.* 2012;110:102–110.

Irvin W, Anderson W, Taylor P, Rice L. Minimizing the risk for neurologic injury in gynecologic surgery. *Obstet Gynecol.* 2004;103(2):374–382.

Nardos R, Browning A, Member B. Duration of bladder catheterization after surgery for obstetric fistula. *Int J Gynaecol Obstet.* 2008;103(e1):30–32.

Wall LL, Arrowsmith SD. The "continence gap": a critical concept in obstetric fistula repair. *Int Urogynecol J Pelvic Floor Dysfunct.* 2007;18:843–844.

Chapter 7
Rectovaginal Fistula and Perineal Lacerations

Erin M. Mellano

GENERAL PRINCIPLES
IMAGING AND OTHER DIAGNOSTICS
PREOPERATIVE PLANNING
SURGICAL MANAGEMENT
PROCEDURES AND TECHNIQUES
    Acute Obstetric Laceration Repairs
    Secondary Closure of a Perineal Wound Breakdown
    Chronic Perineal Laceration Repair
PEARLS AND PITFALLS
POSTOPERATIVE CARE
OUTCOMES
COMPLICATIONS

Rectovaginal Fistula and Perineal Lacerations

Erin M. Mellano

GENERAL PRINCIPLES

Definition

- Rectovaginal fistulas (RVFs) are connections between the bowel and the vagina (Fig. 7.1). Terminology to describe fistulas is typically as follows:
  - RVFs occur above the dentate line.
  - Anovaginal fistulas (AVFs) occur below the dentate line.
  - Fistula-in-ano is a communication between the epithelialized surface of the anal canal and the perineal skin (Fig. 7.2).
  - Colovaginal fistulas occur above the rectum and involve the colon.
- There are several classification systems; however, none have consensus validation. In general these systems are based on location (low, middle, high), complexity, and etiology.
- RVFs are most frequently caused by obstetrical trauma. In developing countries, RVFs are most frequently associated with obstructed labor leading to necrosis of the rectovaginal septum and breakdown of the tissues. In developed nations, obstetric RVF formation is more frequently caused by perineal lacerations or episiotomies that occur at time of vaginal delivery. These wounds are repaired after the delivery and are either inadequately repaired, break down, or become infected. Additional etiologies include complications of surgery, inflammatory bowel disorders, infections (e.g., perirectal abscess), congenital malformations, radiation injury, trauma, and cancer. A contemporary cause is complication from transvaginal mesh placed between the vagina and rectum during prolapse repair.
- Perineal lacerations are classified based on the depth of the laceration and structures disrupted (Fig. 7.3).[1]
  - First-degree laceration: Skin and subcutaneous tissues are disrupted, but perineal muscles are intact.
  - Second-degree laceration: Laceration extends into the fascia and muscles of the perineal body, but anal sphincter complex is intact.
  - Third-degree laceration: Laceration extends and involves the anal sphincter muscles but not into the rectal mucosa.

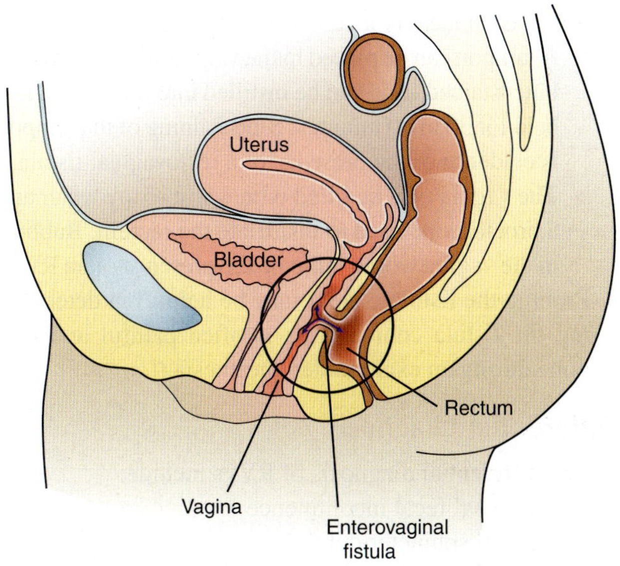

Figure 7.1. Classic rectovaginal fistula. (From Taylor C, Lillis C, Lynn P. *Fundamentals of Nursing*. 8th ed. Philadelphia, PA: Wolters Kluwer; 2014.)

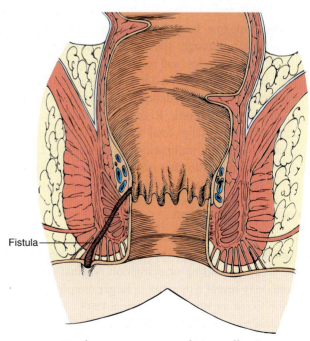

Figure 7.2. Fistula-in-ano. (From Weber J, Kelley J. *Health Assessment in Nursing*. 2nd ed. Philadelphia, PA: Lippincott Williams & Wilkins; 2003.)

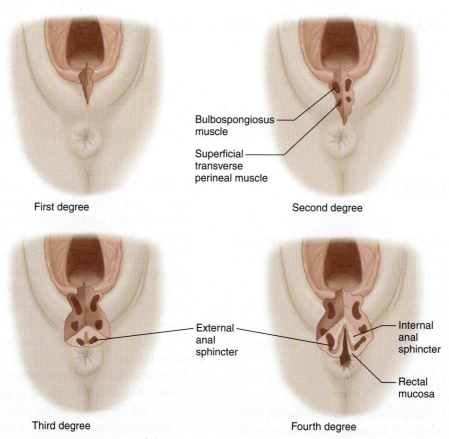

Figure 7.3. Perineal laceration classification.

- 3a: <50% of external anal sphincter (EAS) torn
- 3b: >50% of EAS torn
- 3c: complete EAS and internal anal sphincter (IAS) tear
- Fourth-degree laceration: Laceration extends full thickness through the perineal structures, anal sphincter muscles, and rectal mucosa.
- The classification is rooted in the evaluation of obstetrical injury, as the vast majority of perineal lacerations occur during childbirth. Risk factors for perineal lacerations include large fetal weight, precipitous birth, operative delivery, nulliparity, and episiotomy. Lacerations of the perineum may occur secondary to penetrating or blunt trauma, including straddle-type injuries.

Physical Examination

- General pelvic examination (see Table 5.1).
- An external perineal exam should be performed to look for areas of scarring or disruption. Vaginal speculum exam may reveal a pinpoint or larger dimpling, granulation tissue, or stool in the vaginal vault.
- A digital rectovaginal exam should be performed to assess:
  - Tissue induration.
  - Anal sphincter integrity.
  - Fecal matter expressed through a dimple or scar in the vagina.
- If the integrity of the sphincter is uncertain, endoanal ultrasound should be used in making the determination. Both the anatomy of the EAS as well as the IAS can be assessed by imaging (Fig. 7.4).
- An anoscope can be used to visualize the tract transrectally.
- If the fistula is not readily identified, several techniques are described to identify in ambulatory setting.
  - A tampon can be placed in the vagina and a methylene blue–stained fluid can be instilled into the rectum and held for 30 to 60 minutes. Blue staining of the tampon is evidence of the presence of a rectovaginal fistula.
  - The vagina may be filled with warm soapy water and a proctoscope used to insufflate the rectum. Bubbles in the vagina would indicate the presence of an RVF.[2]
- Probing the fistulous tract may be helpful in determining the fistula course. This is often painful and best done during an exam under anesthesia (Fig. 7.5).

Differential Diagnosis

- The differential diagnosis of RVFs include:
  - Transanal fecal incontinence
    - Anal sphincter defect
    - Anal sphincter neurologic disorder
    - An underlying disease state
  - Perirectal abscess drainage
  - Enterovaginal fistula

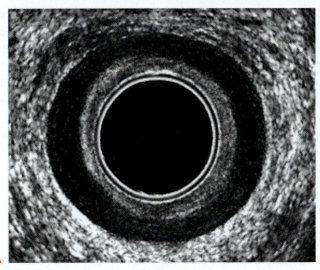 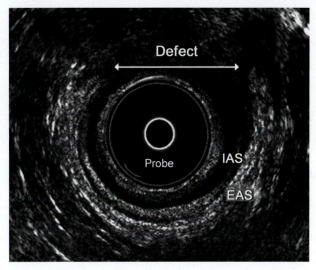

Figure 7.4. Endoanal ultrasound demonstrating anal sphincter ultrastructure. **A:** Intact EAS (hyperechoic ring), intact IAS (hypoechoic ring). **B:** Defect in EAS from 10:00 to 2:00. EAS, external anal sphincter; IAS, internal anal sphincter. (**Part B** courtesy of Justin A. Maykel, MD. In: Jones HW, Rock JA, eds. *Te Linde's Operative Gynecology*. 11th ed. Philadelphia, PA: Wolters Kluwer; 2015.)

Nonoperative Management

- Patients may respond to conservative management alone by preventing diarrhea with diet and stool bulking.
- Up to 50% of small obstetric fistula may heal in the first 6 to 9 months after delivery.
- A seton may be placed to promote healing while awaiting surgical correction. It my be made of thread, wire, rubber, or medicated suture. (Fig. 7.6).
    - A draining seton can be used to help eliminate infection prior to surgical repair.

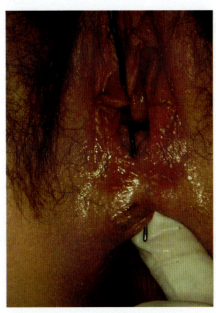

Figure 7.5. Examination of rectovaginal fistula by transvaginal placement of probe through fistula and guidance on finger transrectally. (From Gibbs RS, Karlan BY, Haney AF, Nygaard IE. *Danforth's Obstetrics and Gynecology*. 10th ed. Philadelphia, PA: Wolters Kluwer; 2008.)

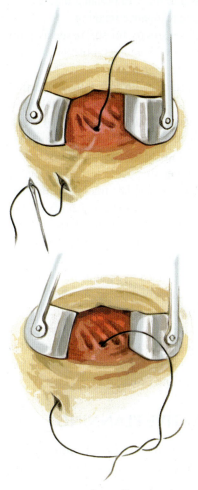

Figure 7.6. Loose seton stitch to allow for drainage of infection while awaiting surgery. (From Wexner SD, Fleshman JW. *Colon and Rectal Surgery: Anorectal Operations*. Philadelphia, PA: Wolters Kluwer; 2011.)

- Cutting setons have been used as alternatives to surgical repair for small perianal fistula.
- Perineal lacerations typically need to be surgically corrected.
- If the underlying cause of fecal incontinence is not related to a fistula, conservative treatment with pelvic floor physical therapy and biofeedback can be helpful in maintaining continence.

IMAGING AND OTHER DIAGNOSTICS

- Diagnostic evaluation may be used when location or presence of the fistula is not definitive on physical exam.
- Contemporary imaging techniques that are helpful in identifying rectal fistulous tracts include:
  - Endoanal or transvaginal ultrasound
    - Adding hydrogen peroxide to highlight the fistulous tract may be required
  - Computed tomography with rectal contrast
    - Most helpful in evaluating perirectal abscesses and inflammation
    - Less helpful with perianal fistulas
  - Magnetic resonance imaging
    - High sensitivity for soft tissue abnormalities
    - Helpful with anorectal fistula
- Other imaging options
  - Fistulography, with insertion of a catheter into the opening of a fistula tract and taking radiographs after injecting radiocontrast media, was a traditional imaging methodology for evaluating fistula tracts. Its utility is limited due to patient discomfort, concerns for disseminating bacteria, and unreliable accuracy.
- Vaginography is another traditional radiographic technique that can be employed to identify the fistulous tract. This technique works best for colovaginal and enterovaginal fistulas, although it has a relatively low sensitivity.
  - A Foley catheter is placed in the vagina and the balloon is expanded to occlude the entrance.
  - Radiopaque contrast is instilled into the vagina through the catheter.
  - X-rays are taken to identify the tract.
- An exam under anesthesia with or without proctoscopy is still considered the definitive method for evaluating the presence and extent of an RVF.

PREOPERATIVE PLANNING

- For patients with RVF, considerations include:
  - The size of the fistula and relationship to the anal sphincter.
  - Tissue integrity and healing phase. Repair should be delayed in the setting of an infection, induration, or severe inflammation.
  - If infection is present, patients should be placed on broad-spectrum antibiotics and surgery delayed until clear. There may be a benefit to a low-residue diet to decrease frequency of stool output.
  - The anal sphincter integrity should be assessed with ultrasonography. It is common for obstetric RVF to have an associated anal sphincter defect.
  - If inflammatory bowel disease is suspected a colonoscopy should be performed.
  - If there is a suspicious mass, biopsies should be performed prior to surgical fistula repair.
  - For patients with prior adjuvant radiation, biopsies should be performed prior to fistula repair to rule out recurrent malignancy.
  - A repair may be approached from the transvaginal or transanal route. If the anal sphincter has been disrupted, a sphincteroplasty should be performed concurrently.
  - Preoperative bowel preparation should be strongly considered to decrease the rate of fecal seeding during the repair and in the immediate postoperative period. The bowel cleansing should begin at least 48 hours before the procedure, and the patient should be on a liquid diet 24 hours prior to the procedure. A rectal enema can be done just before surgery to completely evacuate the rectal vault.
  - For a complex, recurrent, or high-output fistula with extensive inflammation, diverting loop colostomy or ileostomy may be performed to allow for inflammation to resolve. After the fistula is surgically corrected, the diversion may be reversed.
- For patients with perineal lacerations, consider:
  - Whether the laceration is acute, chronic, or from wound breakdown.
  - For patients with acute third- or fourth-degree lacerations, a single dose of broad-spectrum antibiotics should be given.
  - For patients with a laceration repair breakdown and infection, broad-spectrum antibiotics should be administered and repair should not be attempted until the infection has cleared and the tissue appears healthy. Even in the absence of infection, before attempting secondary closure, the necrotic tissue should be debrided until healthy granulation tissue covers the wound.

SURGICAL MANAGEMENT

- The majority of RVFs and perineal lacerations are managed surgically.
- All procedures should be performed in rooms of sufficient size to allow for the surgeon and assistant.

Positioning

- These procedures are typically performed with the patient in the lithotomy position, similar to other gynecologic procedures (see Chapter 5, Tech Fig. 5.18).
  - Various lithotomy stirrups are available to assure patient safety and comfort, minimizing risk for related injury.
  - Arms may be left untucked for easy intravenous access by the anesthesiologist or nurse if needed.

Approach

- The approach to surgical management of **rectovaginal fistula** should focus on the anatomic location of the fistula and relationship to the anal sphincter.
  - If the anal sphincter is intact, a simple fistula repair can be performed.
  - Sphincteroplasty should be performed when the anal sphincter is disrupted.

Transvaginal Approach Without Sphincteroplasty

- This is the traditional gynecologic approach to fistula repair.
- Patients are placed in the dorsal lithotomy position to allow for perineal and vaginal access.
- The fistula tract should be well visualized. A thin probe, such as a lacrimal duct probe, may be placed in the tract to best delineate the course.
- Initial step is to isolate the fistula from the vaginal side. A circumferential incision is made around the fistula opening. Leaving a 2- to 3-mm margin of epithelium around the fistula is acceptable.
- Wide mobilization of the vaginal epithelium off of the underlying rectum and prerectal fascia around the fistulous tract is necessary to facilitate a tension-free repair (Fig. 7.7).
- The full-thickness fistulous tract may then be excised.
- The underlying rectal mucosal defect is then closed in an interrupted fashion using 3.0 or 4.0 delayed absorbable suture.
- A second layer of the same suture is used to reinforce the lateral muscularis layer.
- The pararectal fascia is then approximated to give a third layer of closure using a 2.0 delayed absorbable suture.
- A vascular fat graft, if needed, may be interposed between the rectum and the vagina (See Chapter 6, p. 115).[3]
- The vaginal epithelium is then closed with a 3.0 delayed absorbable suture.

Transvaginal Approach With Sphincteroplasty

- Initially a transverse perineal incision, with cephalad mobilization of the vaginal epithelium and

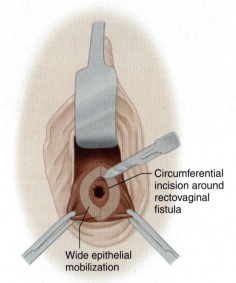

Figure 7.7. Creation of a circumferential incision through vaginal epithelium around fistulous tract.

identification of the sphincter muscles, is performed. The incision should extend to and just above the area of the fistula.
- The rectal mucosal defect is identified and the edges of the fistula are excised and freshened to allow reapproximation of healthy rectal mucosa. The rectal mucosa is then closed using a 3.0 or 4.0 delayed absorbable suture.
- The IAS can be repaired in a running fashion using a 2.0 or 3.0 delayed absorbable suture (Fig. 7.8).
- The EAS may be repaired in two techniques. Both techniques can utilize 2.0 delayed absorbable suture such as polyglactin 910 or longer-lasting delayed absorbable suture like polydioxanone sulfate PDS.
  - End to end: interrupted sutures at 12, 3, 6, and 9 o'clock
  - Overlapping: 2 to 3 mattress sutures (Fig. 7.9)
- Randomized controlled trials have shown no differences in long-term outcomes in end-to-end versus overlapping sphincter repair of the EAS.

Transperineal Approach

- Appropriate approach for fistulas above the anal sphincter.
- Transverse incision made in the perineal body above the sphincter.
- Dissection between the anterior rectal wall and the posterior vaginal wall cephalad and lateral to the fistula tract.
- Scar tissue and devitalized tissue are excised around the fistula tract.

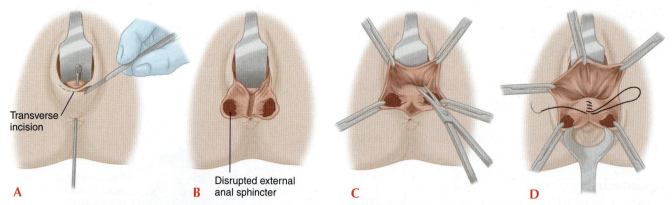

Figure 7.8. A, B: The fistula is identified and a probe is placed to mark the course. A vertical incision is made in the perineal body and extended to the fistula. **C:** The vagina and rectum are separated. **D:** The fistulous tract is excised/mucosal edges are refreshed. The rectal mucosa is closed in a running fashion using 3.0 or 4.0 delayed absorbable suture. (Adapted, courtesy of James L. Breen, MD, Caterina A. Gregori, MD. In: Corman MC, Nicholls RJ, Fazio VW, Bergamaschi R, eds. *Corman's Colon and Rectal Surgery*. 6th ed. Philadelphia, PA: Wolters Kluwer; 2012.)

- The rectal mucosal defect is closed in a tension-free manner using interrupted fashion with 3.0 or 4.0 delayed absorbable suture, taking care to invert the tissue.
- The rectal wall can be closed transversely or longitudinally.
- The muscularis of the rectum is closed in a second layer to reinforce the repair with 2.0 delayed suture in an interrupted fashion.
- The puborectalis muscles are approximated in the midline.
- The vaginal epithelium is closed in a running fashion with 2.0 or 3.0 delayed absorbable suture.
- The subcutaneous tissue and skin of the perineal body are approximated.
- The perineal skin is closed with 4.0 delayed absorbable suture. It can either be closed in a subcutaneous fashion or with interrupted mattress sutures.

Interposition of a Neovascular Tissue Flap

- Interposition of a neovascular flap is helpful when there are concerns for poor healing, such as:
  - Complex fistulas
  - Radiation fistulas
  - Prior failed fistula repairs
  - Devitalized tissue or decreased vascularity
- Martius or fat pad graft
  - This is an easily accessible source of vascularized tissue for distal to mid-vaginal fistulas. Blood supply to the Martius flap is derived from the external pudendal artery superiorly and from the internal pudendal artery inferiorly. Lateral blood supply is derived from the obturator artery (Fig. 7.10).
  - The patient must have adequate labial fat for this to be a possible procedure.
  - The primary closure of the RVF is as described above with traditional fistula repair until the point of closing the vaginal epithelium.
  - The Martius graft is harvested from the right or left labia majora. Choice of side should depend on the patient's anatomy and fistula location.
  - A 6- to 8-cm incision is made over the labia majora, and sharp dissection is used to mobilize the bulbocavernosus fat pad. Dissection is carried down to the fascia (Fig. 7.11).
  - Superiorly, the external pudendal artery is ligated and transected, leaving a broad fat pad base with intact blood supply from the branch of the internal pudendal artery.
  - An incision is then made in the wall of the vagina to allow for transfer of the graft into the vagina. A tunnel is created to allow for passage of the graft to the fistula site.

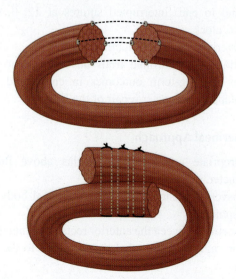

- **Figure 7.9.** Anal sphincteroplasty techniques. **Upper:** End-to-end repair. **Lower:** Overlapping.

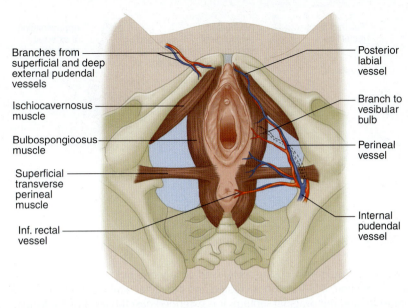

Figure 7.10. Blood supply to the fatty tissue for Martius graft transposition is from internal pudendal artery dorsally and from external pudendal artery ventrally.

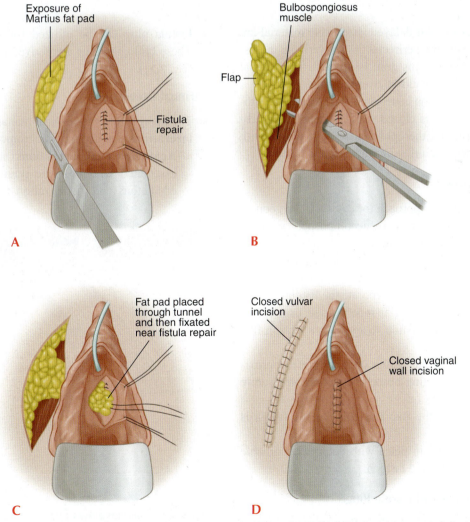

Figure 7.11. A: Creation of Martius flap begins with a longitudinal incision over the labia majora. **B:** Mobilization of the labial fat and ligation of the corresponding pudendal blood supply. **C:** Transfer of the flap to the vaginal wound and fixation over repaired fistula. **D:** Closure of both wounds.

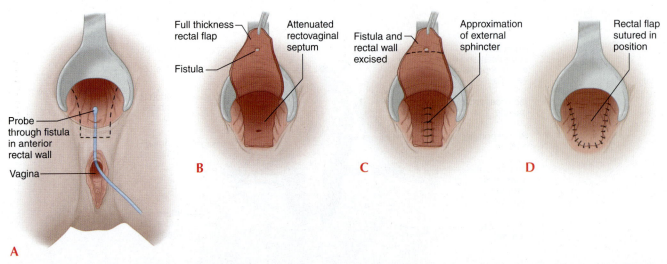

Figure 7.12. Transanal rectovaginal fistula repair using rectal wall advancement. **A:** The patient is shown placed in the **PRONE** position. **B:** Starting at the dentate line, a U-incision is created and the rectal wall is mobilized in a cephalad direction from the underlying sphincter muscles and rectovaginal septum. It is extended past the level of the fistula. **C:** The rectovaginal wall is plicated and spinchteric unit is reinforced if disrupted. **D:** The mobilized rectal wall flap is advanced over the rectal wall and closed with interrupted sutures. (Adapted from Michelassi F. Crohn's disease. In: Bell RH Jr, Rikkers LF, Mulholland MW, eds. *Digestive Tract Surgery: A Text and Atlas*. Philadelphia, PA: Lippincott-Raven; 1996:1201.)

- Stay sutures of 2.0 delayed absorbable material are placed around the perirectal tissue overlying the fistula, and the Martius graft is secured. The vaginal epithelium is then closed over the graft.
- The vulvar incision is irrigated and closed. The subcutaneous layer is closed with 2.0 delayed absorbable suture, and the epithelial layer is closed with 4.0 Monocryl in a running subcuticular fashion.

Transanal Approach (Fig. 7.12)[4]

- This is a traditional approach for colorectal surgeons.
- For simple fistula, this is accomplished with an endorectal advancement flap.
- The patient is placed in a prone jackknife position.
- A probe is placed through the fistula to identify the tract.
- A U incision is made to incorporate the fistula.
- Wide mobilization of the flap is performed, usually 4 to 5 cm cephalad to the fistula, to allow for a tension-free repair.
- The muscles over the fistula opening are reapproximated with long-acting absorbable interrupted suture in two layers.
- The distal end of the flap that contains the fistula is excised.
- The flap is sutured in place with delayed absorbable suture in an interrupted fashion.

Fistula Fibrin Glue and Fistula Plugs

- Fibrin glue has a limited role in fistula repair. Success rates are between 10% and 64% for cryptoglandular anal fistulas.
- Fistula plug can be utilized for small <1 cm RVF. These biologic plugs are derived from animal sources (**Fig. 7.13**).

Perineal Lacerations

- The approach to the surgical management of **perineal lacerations** will depend on chronicity of the defect.
  - **Acute perineal lacerations** are most frequently associated with obstetric trauma. Tissue is often edematous and visualization may be complicated

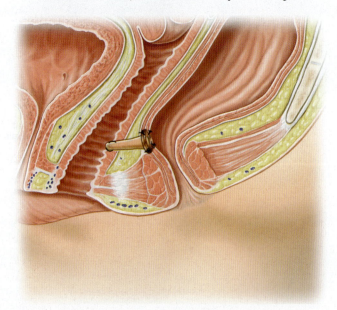

Figure 7.13. Sagittal view of fistula plug anchored transrectally. (From Wexner SD, Fleshman JW. *Colon and Rectal Surgery: Anorectal Operations*. Philadelphia, PA: Wolters Kluwer; 2011.)

by uterine bleeding. It is best to wait until after delivery of the placenta. This will allow for better visualization and eliminates the risk for disturbing your repair at the time of removal. Ensure that there is good uterine tone to minimize uterine bleeding into the field and that all lacerations cephalad to the perineum have been repaired. The degree of laceration should be assessed and this will dictate the type of repair. Regardless of the depth of the laceration, it is important to make sure that there is adequate anesthesia—either with the epidural or local infiltration of anesthetic. Proper lighting and instrumentation are essential, as optimizing surgical conditions will produce optimal results for the patient.

- **Perineal wound breakdown** can occur in the first week or two after repair. The wound should be evaluated for infection, and if present, antibiotics given. The tissues should be inspected and debrided until healthy pink granulation tissue covers the surface of the wound. Sitz baths can be done for patient comfort and to keep the area clean. Once devitalized tissue is absent and infection clears, the wound can be repaired under sterile conditions.
- **Chronic or old perineal lacerations** are approached in a slightly different manner. The tissues are typically not edematous, but scarring can be significant and tissue planes need to be developed to allow for proper closure.

Acute Obstetric Laceration Repairs

First- and Second-Degree Lacerations

- These are typically repaired with a 2.0 or 3.0 delayed absorbable suture in a running fashion. The repair starts at the most cephalad point of the laceration in the vaginal canal and is run continuously until the hymenal ring is reached and reapproximated. The suture is then redirected to repair the muscles of the bulbospongiosus and transverse perineal muscles in a caudal direction. The continuous suture is then used to close the skin in a subcuticular fashion with the final suture and knot placed behind the hymenal ring.

Third-Degree Lacerations

- A single dose of broad-spectrum antibiotics is recommended.
- These closures should be initiated with identification of the degree of involvement of the anal sphincter. Adequate visualization and anesthesia are paramount. There may be a role for repair in the operating room if these cannot be achieved in the labor and delivery suite.
- If the anal sphincter is completely disrupted, the IAS may have retracted laterally and need to be dissected free to allow for mobilization to bring it back to the midline. If the IAS was disrupted, it should be repaired in a running fashion using 2.0 or 3.0 delayed absorbable suture.
- The EAS is repaired in an interrupted figure-of-eight fashion at 12, 3, 6, and 9 o'clock using 2.0 delayed absorbable suture. The mnemonic "PISA" (Posterior, Inferior, Superior, Anterior) is often used to describe the order of suture placement in repairing the EAS.
    - Randomized controlled trials have shown no differences in long-term outcomes in end-to-end versus overlapping sphincter repair of the EAS.
- The remainder of the closure is approached in the same way as described above for second-degree lacerations.

Fourth-Degree Lacerations

- Similar to third-degree lacerations, a single dose of broad-spectrum antibiotics is recommended (**Tech Fig. 7.1**).
- These wounds are characterized by involvement of the rectal mucosa. The mucosa is identified and 3.0 or 4.0 delayed absorbable suture is used to reapproximate the mucosa.
- A reinforcing suture line incorporating the IAS is also accomplished with a continuous 3.0 or 4.0 suture.
- The remainder of the closure is approached in the same fashion as described above for third-degree lacerations.

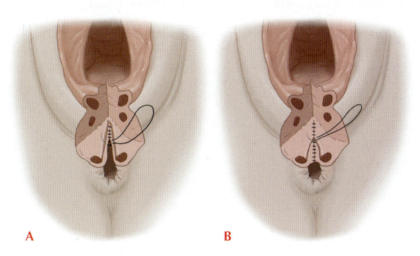

A **B**

Tech Figure 7.1. Repair of fourth-degree laceration is best done in layers with separate sutures.

Secondary Closure of a Perineal Wound Breakdown

- All signs of infections should have resolved and healthy tissue edges should be present prior to attempting secondary repair of a perineal laceration.
- Preoperative antibiotics are often given with a broad-spectrum cephalosporin. If the wound involves the anal sphincter or mucosa, anaerobic coverage with metronidazole should be added.
- The wound is repaired in the same fashion as an acute laceration; however, there may be a role for interrupted sutures to help reinforce integrity of the repair.

Chronic Perineal Laceration Repair

- The patient is placed in dorsal lithotomy position after regional or general anesthesia has been administered (**Tech Fig. 7.2**).

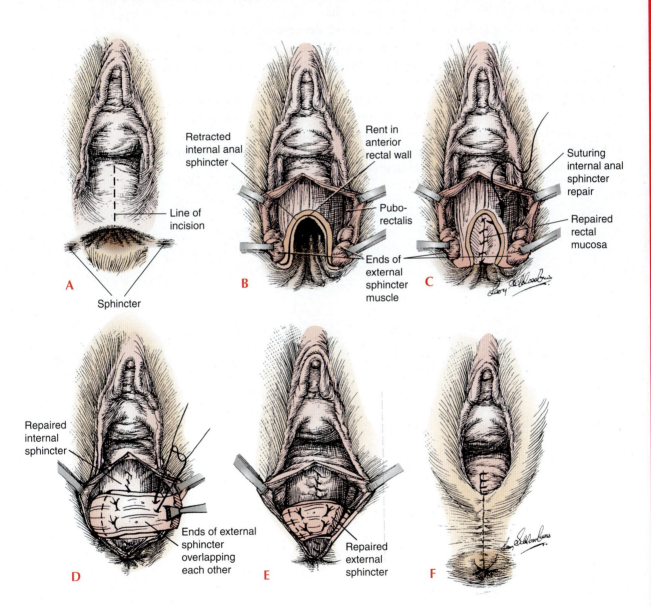

Tech Figure 7.2. Repair of chronic perineal laceration. (From Jones HW, Rock JA, eds. *Te Linde's Operative Gynecology*. 11th ed. Philadelphia, PA: Wolters Kluwer; 2015.)

- A transverse incision is made at the rectal mucosal–vaginal epithelial junction, and the tissues are separated using sharp dissection.
- The EAS has typically retracted laterally and needs to be identified. Once identified, Allis clamps are used to grasp the ends, and they are dissected sufficiently to allow for mobilization to the midline. Dissection should not be carried out further than 3 o'clock and 9 o'clock to avoid injury to nerves to the anus.
- The IAS is a fibrinous layer between the rectal mucosa and the EAS.
- The repair is initiated by approximating the dissected free rectal mucosa using a 3.0 or 4.0 delayed absorbable suture in a running fashion. This layer is reinforced with repair of the IAS in a running fashion using a 3.0 delayed absorbable suture.
- Attention is then turned to the EAS. Once adequately mobilized with sharp dissection, it is repaired in an end-to-end or overlapping fashion with rows of 2.0 delayed absorbable or permanent horizontal mattress sutures.
- The genital hiatus is narrowed by bringing the puborectalis muscles closer together.
- The bulbospongiosus muscles and transverse perineal muscles are reapproximated in an interrupted fashion with 2.0 delayed absorbable suture.
- The vaginal epithelium is closed with 2.0 or 3.0 delayed absorbable suture in a running fashion similar to a first- or second-degree perineal laceration.

PEARLS AND PITFALLS

DIAGNOSIS OF RVF

- Physical exam can be definitive. For a small fistula, examination under anesthesia may be required. Endoanal ultrasound can be utilized to assess anal sphincter integrity.

TIMING OF REPAIR

- Repair should be performed in the absence of infection and severe inflammation. Early repair is possible if there is limited induration and inflammation. If in doubt delay repair until conditions are optimized.

REPAIR TECHNIQUE

- RVF can be repaired transvaginally or transanally. Most distal to mid RVF can be done via the transvaginal route. If location is juxtasphincteric or not easily accessible transvaginally, then transrectal with rectal flap advancement may be preferred.

PERINEAL LACERATION

- Identification of the extent of injury and presence of sphincter or rectal wall involvement is critical during diagnosis. Appropriate repair can be selected to avoid fecal incontinence or future fistula formation.

POSTREPAIR PERINEAL CARE

- Proper perineal care with constipation and straining avoidance as well as perineal hygiene are important to avoid incisional complications and wound breakdown.

POSTOPERATIVE CARE

- Postrepair perineal care is similar for all types of laceration repairs.
  - Stools should be kept soft to avoid constipation. Laxatives can be added to the regimen as needed.
  - Analgesia with nonsteroidal anti-inflammatory (NSAIDs) medications rather than narcotics. NSAIDs are generally well tolerated, assist in decreasing inflammation, and have fewer unwanted side effects.
  - Topical anesthetics can be used to decrease discomfort, although data suggest that there is no improvement over placebo.
  - Cold compresses or ice packs can be helpful to decrease swelling.
  - Sitz baths can also be used for symptom relief.
- Implementation and timing of pelvic floor physical therapy should be done with careful consideration. In general, healing should be complete prior to initiation of any pelvic floor muscle rehabilitation.

OUTCOMES

- For RVF, repair outcomes are generally high above 80% for non-cancer or inflammatory bowel–related diseases. Rates of incontinence to flatus or stool are higher when sphincteric injury is associated.
- For obstetrical anal sphincter laceration the data available show that at 1-year follow-up, immediate primary overlap repair of the EAS compared with immediate primary end-to-end repair appears to be associated with lower risks of developing fecal urgency and anal incontinence symptoms. At the end of 36 months there appears to be no difference in flatus or fecal incontinence between the two techniques. However, since this evidence is based on only two small trials, more research evidence is needed in order to confirm or refute these findings.

COMPLICATIONS

- Complications after RVF repair are generally low, with wound infections being highest when there are associated perineal lacerations.
- Recurrence rates are between 7% and 19% requiring additional surgery.
- Mortality is exceedingly rare.

KEY REFERENCES

1. Sultan AH. Obstetric perineal injury and anal incontinence (editorial). *Clin Risk.* 1999;5:193–196.
2. Lowry AC, Hoexter B. Benign anorectal: Rectovaginal fistulas. In: Steele SR, Hull TL, Read ThE, Saclarides TJ, Senagore AJ, Whitlow CB (Eds), *The ASCRS Textbook of Colon and Rectal Surgery.* New York: Springer; 2007:215–227.
3. Eilber KS, Kavaler E, Rodriguez LV, et al. Ten-year experience with transvaginal vesicovaginal fistula repair using tissue interposition. *J Urol.* 2003;169:1033–1036.
4. Fernando R, Sultan AH, Kettle C, Thakar R. Methods of repair for obstetric anal sphincter injury. *Cochrane Database Syst Rev.* 2013;(12): CD002866.
5. Royal College of Obstetricians and Gynaecologists. Green-top guideline no. 29: The management of third- and fourth-degree perineal tears. March 2007. https://www.rcog.org.uk/en/guidelines-research-services/guidelines/gtg29/
6. Dudding TC, Vaizey CJ, Kamm MA. Obstetric anal sphincter injury: incidence, risk factors, and management. *Ann Surg.* 2008;247:224.

Chapter 8
Approach to Removal of Vaginal Mesh

Lisa Rogo-Gupta

GENERAL PRINCIPLES
IMAGING AND OTHER DIAGNOSTICS
PREOPERATIVE PLANNING
SURGICAL MANAGEMENT
PROCEDURES AND TECHNIQUES
    Removal of Vaginal Mesh
    Technique
PEARLS AND PITFALLS
POSTOPERATIVE CARE
OUTCOMES
COMPLICATIONS

Approach to Removal of Vaginal Mesh
Lisa Rogo-Gupta

GENERAL PRINCIPLES

Definition
- Surgical correction of symptomatic pelvic organ prolapse (POP) or urinary incontinence (UI) may be performed using a variety of methods. The traditional repair technique for prolapse of the vaginal walls, known as colporrhaphy, has been the mainstay for correcting vaginal prolapse for decades. The colporrhaphy when done for anterior prolapse or *cystocele* has been termed anterior repair and when done for posterior prolapse or *rectocele* termed posterior repair. With the advent of synthetic mesh, that took hold in the early and mid-2000s, traditional repairs were termed *native tissue* repairs to distinguish them from repairs that utilized additional materials or *augmented* repairs. Use of allografts, xenografts, or synthetic material, such as mesh, has been added to vaginal repairs by surgeons in hope of improving the durability or longevity of the repair.
- The term "mesh" commonly refers to a synthetic graft used to augment POP or UI repairs.
  - Polypropylene is the most commonly used synthetic material for such grafts. Many commercially available products have been introduced and/or removed from the marketplace; thus this chapter will focus on general surgical techniques that may be applied to removal of grafts in general.
  - Mid-urethral slings are considered standard care for uncomplicated stress urinary incontinence (SUI).
  - Mesh can be placed vaginally or abdominally for POP repair of the anterior, apical, or posterior compartments. It is critical to differentiate the route of placement, vaginal versus abdominal, when analyzing and considering mesh-augmented prolapse surgery. For the purpose of this chapter we will focus on *vaginal* route of mesh placement.

Physical Examination
- General pelvic examination (see Chapter 5, **Table 5.1**).
- The evaluation and management of women with symptoms occurring after mesh-augmented vaginal surgery for prolapse and incontinence has been one of the most challenging issues facing pelvic reconstructive surgeons in the last decade.
- For patients with **possible mesh-related complications**, these additional steps should be considered:
  - A discriminate vaginal and pelvic exam is vital. Patients with mesh-related pain often present in a state of true pelvic floor *dysfunction*. Identifying and understanding the anatomy, the actual location of the mesh, and the associated myofascial and visceral dysfunction are crucial. Identifying and distinguishing the presence of pain generators, scarring, and trigger points will facilitate a cogent management approach (see **Pearls and Pitfalls**).
  - Palpate perineal and introital structures. Discern introital caliber by gentle dual digital distension, as a source for dyspareunia.
  - Palpate levator ani, specifically the hiatus of the pubococcygeus to determine resting state, presence of allodynia, and ability to contract and relax.
  - Palpate along the path of the implant, both expected and actual.
  - Identify discrepancies between expected location of placement and actual location. This is essential for decision making regarding partial versus complete excision as well as for incision planning.
  - Identify areas of folding, tines, or other attachment devices.
  - Explore for vaginal exposure, which often is asymptomatic. This is often most easily done via palpation, as small exposures may be difficult to visualize.
  - Document areas of pain or tenderness.
  - Visualize skin exit sites (see **Pearls and Pitfalls**).
  - Evaluate the quality and quantity of vaginal epithelium. This is essential for preoperative planning in cases where flaps must be created for a tension-free closure over defects.
  - Documentation of mesh-related complications can be performed using a standard system designed to facilitate common nomenclature among physicians. However, this system is not all-inclusive and a narrative report of subjective complaints and objective findings

is recommended. Using the hymen as a reference point is helpful in documenting and measuring location of any exposures.
- Post-void residual (PVR) is the measurement of urine in the bladder following urination by transabdominal ultrasound or by catheterization. PVR assessment should be performed in patients with symptoms suggestive of partial or complete obstruction.
- Urinalysis or culture should be performed to rule out urinary tract infection in patients with symptoms suggestive of infection.
- Cystoscopy should be performed to exclude erosion into the bladder or urethra in suspect cases.

Differential Diagnosis

- Patients with a history of POP or UI mesh placement who present with symptoms should be carefully evaluated as to whether or not the symptoms are likely secondary to the mesh grafts.
  - For example, urge UI occurs in 6% of women who undergo synthetic mid-urethral slings and persists in 44% of those with pre-existing symptoms. The presence of this symptom postoperatively should not alone be considered a reason for mesh excision. The patient's overall clinical picture should be considered and the patient is offered conservative management unless other signs of urinary obstruction are present.
  - Urinary retention lasting more than 30 days or requiring intervention is an example of a complication of synthetic mid-urethral slings that occurs in approximately 3% of cases. There is no consensus on the performance of sling incision versus partial excision for the indication of urinary retention. Both can be considered in the management for this sequela.
- The differential diagnosis for each presenting symptom should be considered as well as the following details:
  - Time of symptom onset in relation to mesh placement
  - Relationship of symptoms to the function of surrounding organs (i.e., urination, defecation, intercourse)
  - Prior treatment for symptoms
  - Impact of symptoms on quality of life
- Mesh removal should be considered early for patients whose symptoms are refractory to conservative and medical management and negatively impacting their overall quality of life.
- Mesh removal surgery is required for any of the following:
  - Visceral erosion.
  - Vaginal exposures that are symptomatic for the patient or partner and are >1 cm, or those that are smaller and do not heal after revision/vaginal estrogen (Fig. 8.1).

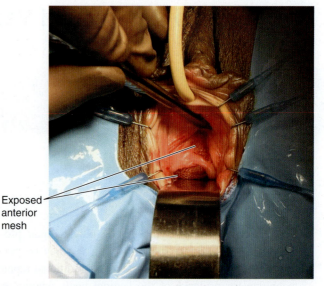

Figure 8.1. Mesh exposure from anterior vaginal mesh.

Nonoperative Management

- Mesh exposure
  - **Vaginal**
    - Conservative management is considered first-line treatment, particularly if small, <1 cm
      - Topical hormone therapy
      - Treatment of active infections
- Pain or dyspareunia
  - Oral or topical medications: Elavil, Gabapentin, Nonsteroidal anti-inflammatory
  - For pelvic pain refractive to conservative treatment. Often pelvic floor physical therapy will not be effective if mesh banding and scarring are present.
  - Pelvic floor physical therapy: soft tissue mobilization, levator ani relaxation
  - Trigger point injections
- Lower urinary tract symptoms
  - Conservative management is considered first-line treatment
    - Anticholinergic therapy for urgency or urge UI
    - Treatment of active infections
- Urinary retention
  - Continuous indwelling catheter
  - Clean intermittent self-catheterization
  - Consideration of surgical management if symptoms do not improve

IMAGING AND OTHER DIAGNOSTICS

- Diagnostic evaluation may be useful when additional information might impact patient counseling and treatment planning. For example, in cases where initial history and examination are inconsistent or inconclusive and a clear diagnosis is not obtained.

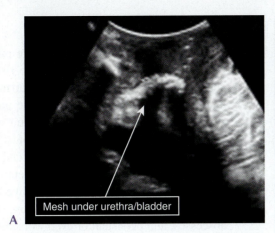
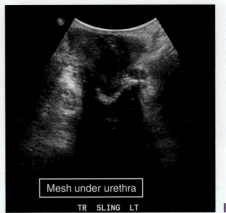

Figure 8.2. Transperineal mesh ultrasound. **A:** Sagittal view. Mesh segment is hyperechoic. **B:** Coronal view of mesh exposure.

- Diagnostic evaluation may include one or more of the following:
  - Ultrasound can be used to visualize mesh and may be useful in cases where graft location is unknown or when multiple revisions have been performed previously (Fig. 8.2).
  - A bladder diary, or frequency–volume chart, is a record of liquid intake, urinary output, and UI of at least one consecutive 24-hour period. This information can be helpful to establish an objective baseline and for the clinician to understand exacerbating factors, symptom severity, and impact on activities of daily living.
  - Urodynamics to evaluate bladder filling, storage, and emptying. Tests may include PVR, cystometry, uroflowmetry, pressure flow studies, video (x-ray) studies, electromyography, and/or urethral function tests. Urodynamics may be performed in patients considering surgical management.
  - Pelvic imaging such as CT scan or MRI may be used in cases where hematoma, abscess, neuroma, neuritis, osteitis, or organ obstruction is suspected. Grafts are typically not clearly seen in these types of studies.
  - Voiding cystourethrogram (VCUG) or vaginal tampon test may be used when urethrovaginal or vesicovaginal fistula is suspected. Urogram or intravenous pyelogram (IVP) is appropriate for suspected ureterovaginal fistula.
  - Contrast enemas or endoanal ultrasound may be used for suspected rectovaginal fistula.

PREOPERATIVE PLANNING

- The goal of surgical mesh removal is to improve quality of life. Preoperative planning begins with an overall assessment of the patient's reported symptoms, objective findings, and most importantly, treatment goals. Understanding of risks, benefits, and treatment alternatives as well as physical capacity to manage unexpected outcomes is essential.
- Office cystoscopy may be considered prior to surgical management to evaluate for erosion into the bladder or urethra. Symptoms suggestive of this complication include recurrent infections, hematuria, dysuria, and lower urinary tract symptoms.
- Proctoscopy may be considered prior to surgical management to evaluate for erosion in the rectum or anus. Symptoms suggestive of this complication include hematochezia, pain with defecation, and fecal urgency.
- For patients with mesh complications, consider:
  - Discussion and documentation of attempts at nonsurgical management prior to surgical management.
  - Age, activity level, and need for possible repeat treatment when considering surgical treatment options.
  - Physical ability and willingness to use pads in cases of postoperative UI, and pessary in cases of postoperative POP.
  - Informed consent regarding the possible short- and long-term complications including hemorrhage, pain, recurrent UI, recurrent exposure, recurrence of prolapse or nonresolution of symptoms.
  - As pain and debility are often the driving symptoms for surgical correction, the goal of surgery should be to optimize chance for resolution of pain. Therefore, concomitant prolapse and/or UI repair should remain a secondary goal. A phased or staged approach is encouraged as patients have potential for maintenance of vaginal support and continence even in light of complete mesh removal.
- **Partial mesh excision and revision** should be considered in these scenarios:
  - Focal vaginal exposure

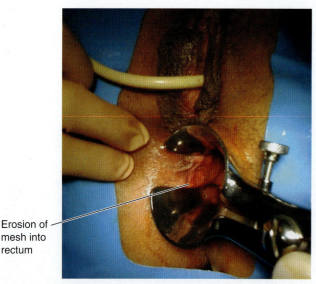

Erosion of mesh into rectum

Figure 8.3. Erosion of mesh into rectum.

- Strong desire to maintain durability of initial procedure for maintenance of prolapse or continence
- Absence of exposure into surrounding organs
- Mild impact on overall quality of life
- **Complete excision** of mesh should be considered in these scenarios:
  - Large vaginal exposure
  - Presence of recurrent infections or severe pain and debility
  - Erosion into surrounding organs (**Fig. 8.3**)
  - Severe impact on overall quality of life
  - Failed other management strategies
  - Belief that mesh is related to global or systemic constitutional symptoms

SURGICAL MANAGEMENT

- The surgical management options are partial excision or total mesh removal. Perioperative risks are varied and are dependent on the extent of scarring present and amount of mesh to be removed. The nature of these cases is such that each is unique and complications are difficult to predict. This type of surgery can be extremely tedious, time consuming, and complicated, particularly with total vaginal mesh removal. Reported complications include acute or delayed hemorrhage requiring transfusion, visceral injury, infections or abscesses, and persistent or even worsening pain.

Positioning

- Vaginal mesh removal procedures are performed with the patient in the lithotomy position, the same position used for placement (see Chapter 2, **Figure 2.4**).
  - Various lithotomy stirrups are available to assure patient safety and comfort, minimizing risk for related injury.
  - Arms may be left untucked for easy intravenous access by the anesthesiologist or nurse, if needed.
- The surgical field should include corresponding locations of mesh arms exit sites, such as the perineum over the obturator foramen, perianal area, or suprapubic area. This will facilitate identification of the mesh in its entirety for cases of complete excision.

Approach

- The approach to mesh removal should focus on overall impact of symptoms on quality of life. Assessment of bother due to symptoms is essential to the discussion of treatment options. Clear understanding of treatment goals and expectations will improve patient satisfaction.

Removal of Vaginal Mesh

- Operative reports should be reviewed preoperatively for details regarding graft type and placement technique.
- The patient is placed on the operating table in the dorsal lithotomy position.
- The approach to excision and revision is generally similar for urinary incontinence (UI) and pelvic organ prolapse (POP) grafts, with some specific considerations depending upon implant type.

Partial Excision of Mesh

- In cases of partial excision, only a portion of the mesh is removed and the vagina is closed over the defect.
- Local anesthetic may be injected into the vagina at the site of the exposed portion(s). Injection of larger volumes is often used to hydrodissect the proper tissue plane and facilitate entry. Commonly used preparations include bupivacaine 0.25% with or without epinephrine, dilute vasopressin, and normal saline 0.9%.
- Using sharp, narrow-tipped scissors such as Metzenbaum scissors, the vaginal wall is undermined circumferentially and widely around the exposed portion for a tension-free closure.
- The exposed mesh portion is excised and removed. The mobilized vagina is then closed over the defect. Close inspection of the vaginal edges should be done to ensure no mesh in the area of the closure. Interrupted absorbable sutures are often used for this purpose.
- Generous irrigation of the wound and defect should be performed prior to closure.
- Careful handling of vaginal epithelium is critical for complication-free closure and success of repair. The edges should be free of macerated or devitalized epithelium. Wide mobilization of the vaginal flap is important to create a tension-free closure **(see Pearls and Pitfalls)**.

Complete Excision

- Technique may vary depending on mesh type and location.
- Local anesthetic may be injected into the vagina at the site of planned entry. Injection of larger volumes is often used to hydrodissect the proper tissue plane and facilitate entry. Commonly used preparations include bupivacaine 0.25% with or without epinephrine, dilute vasopressin, and normal saline 0.9%.

Incision Planning

- For either a mid-urethral sling or a **POP mesh removal**, a vertical or an inverted-U incision is made in the covering vaginal wall, with careful planning to allow access laterally for removal as well as a tension-free closure upon completion (**Tech Fig. 8.1**; **Video 8.1**).

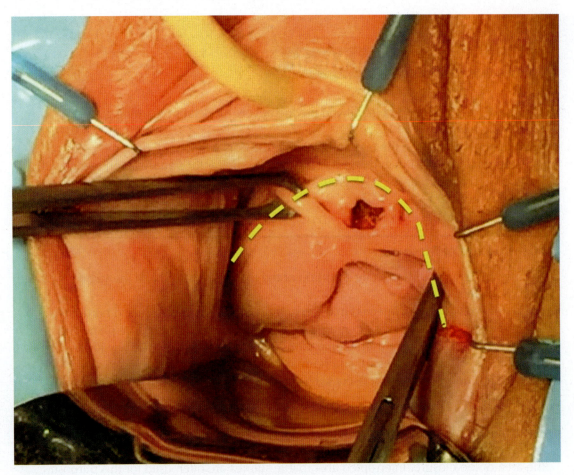

Tech Figure 8.1. Location of inverted-U incision for the removal of transvaginal mesh or sling.

- A combination of sharp and blunt dissection is used to free the vagina from the mesh laterally to isolate the implant arms or fixation devices in appropriate cases.
- The goal should be to mobilize the vaginal epithelium off of the underlying mesh. The vaginal epithelium should be mobilized widely off of the mesh to ensure mesh removal and to allow proper closure.
- Care should be used to avoid incising the mesh prior to epithelial mobilization.
- In some instances, mesh separation from the vaginal wall may be challenging or impossible as the mesh can be intimately integrated into the vaginal wall. This is a consequence of scarring or split-thickness technique when implant is performed. Removal of mesh-impregnated epithelium should be done, and tissue flap techniques employed to properly close the vagina and preserve function.
- Any vaginal wall imbedded with mesh must be excised.

Technique

- Dissecting laterally toward the ischiopubic rami should be performed.
- Entering the retropubic space between the mesh and the bone will help facilitate the rest of the dissection and should be achieved prior to proceeding with mesh removal (**Video 8.2** ▶).
- For mid-urethral sling, after the central portion of the mesh is exposed, a right-angle clamp can be carefully placed between the mesh and the urethra. Placing the clamp just lateral to the midline can reduce risk of urethral injury (**Video 8.3** ▶).
- The right-angle clamp can be inserted to facilitate separation from the underlying organ(s) using gentle traction (see **Pearls and Pitfalls**).
- With the central portion exposed, the mesh can then be bisected. Using a tonsil clamp on the edge, ipsilateral dissection can be performed laterally. Remove the mesh using gentle traction and Metzenbaum dissection.
- For POP mesh, central exposure is also preferable. The mesh can be mobilized off of underlying bladder or rectum.
- *Incision of the mesh into multiple small pieces is not recommended.*
- Removal of arms can be challenging. Similar to sling mesh removal, a key step to facilitating removal is to bisect the mesh in the midline. Then tension applied to the cut ends of the central portion can be used to follow the arms laterally to their points of attachment or exit. The surrounding tissue is separated from the graft using careful sharp and blunt dissection. Caution should be taken with sharp dissection as arms may traverse in close proximity to the neurovasculature.
  - Alternatively, in cases of skin exit sites, small puncture incisions can be made in the skin and the distal end of the arm identified. Using gentle traction, for example, with an Allis or a tonsil clamp, the mesh is followed proximally and carefully separated from the surrounding tissues.
- The graft is then removed from the patient in its entirety (**Tech Fig. 8.2**).

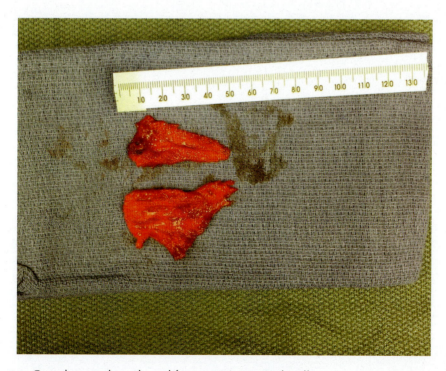

Tech Figure 8.2. Complete mesh explanted from anterior vaginal wall.

- With the mesh completely removed (**Tech Fig. 8.3**) remnant prolapse can be repaired with a modest native tissue repair to reinforce the vaginal walls (see Chapters 1 and 3).
- The vaginal wall is then closed using absorbable sutures in either running or interrupted fashion.

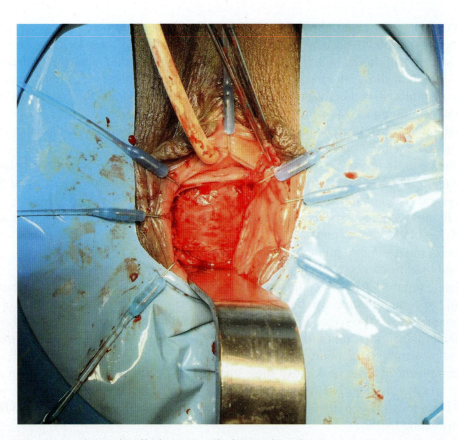

Tech Figure 8.3. Anterior vaginal wall after removal of vaginal mesh.

Retropubic Arm Removal

- Once the central mesh portion is dissected laterally and the retropubic space is reached, the arms can be successfully removed. The retropubic space is entered vaginally by perforating the endopelvic fascia at the location of the sling arm using scissors. The mesh arm is released from the posterior pubic bone and perivesical tissues, and gentle traction then reveals the location of attachment to the anterior abdominal wall. This attachment may be transected through the retropubic space or through a suprapubic skin incision.

Transobturator Arm Removal

- The obturator fascia and obturator internus are perforated sharply at the location of mesh perforation. The arm is then carefully dissected off the pubic bone, obturator membrane, and obturator externus, and gentle traction reveals the location as it traverses the adductor fossa toward the lateral labial or medial thigh exit site. A skin incision can be made at the exit site, which will reveal the underlying adductor fascia, gracilis, and adductor longus muscles. The implant is separated from these structures and transferred through the adductor fossa for removal (**Tech Fig. 8.4**).
- In all cases, once the implant has been removed, cystoscopy should be performed to confirm no bladder perforation has occurred.
- The skin incisions are then closed using absorbable sutures or skin adhesive and covered with dressings. Vaginal packing can be placed for local compression in cases of significant dissection or when bleeding is a concern.

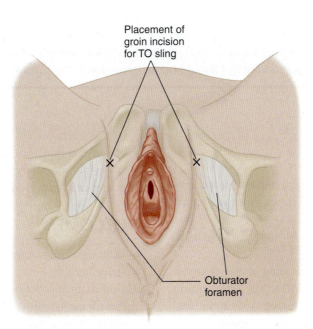

Tech Figure 8.4. Obturator foramen anatomy.

PEARLS AND PITFALLS

BLADDER LANDMARKS

- When concerned about bladder injury during mesh removal, the bladder can be filled with sterile saline stained with dye such as methylene blue. Injury then results in outflow of blue fluid. This facilitates immediate recognition and repair.

DISCRIMINATE PELVIC EXAM

- Identifying and understanding the anatomy, the actual location of the mesh, and the associated myofascial and visceral dysfunction is crucial. Palpate perineal and introital structures. Discern introital caliber by gentle dual digital distension as a source for dyspareunia. Palpate levator ani, specifically the hiatus of the pubococcygeus to determine resting state, presence of allodynia, and ability to contract and relax.

SKIN LANDMARKS

- Small skin scars can often be seen with close examination at the location of prior trocar puncture sites. Overlying hair must often be removed to facilitate visualization. If scars cannot be visualized, an alternate identification method is to place gentle tension on the mesh vaginally. The skin can then be seen to pucker inward at the location of the puncture.

HANDLING OF VAGINAL TISSUE

- Careful handling of vaginal epithelium is critical for complication-free closure and success of excision repair. The edges should be free of macerated or devitalized epithelium. Wide mobilization of the vaginal flap is important to create a tension-free closure. Generous irrigation of the wound and defect should be performed prior to closure.

POSTOPERATIVE CARE

- Postoperative care following mesh removal procedures is similar to that for other benign urogynecologic surgeries (see Chapter 5, Table 5.6).
- Antibiotics are **recommended** for the following mesh removal procedures:
    - Vaginal prolapse mesh and sling mesh removal: Guidelines from the surgical care improvement project (SCIP) recommend using a first- or second-generation cephalosporin for 24 hours.
- Continuous bladder drainage after mesh removal surgery is only required when there is a transgression of the bladder or urethra. Other instances for prolonged bladder drainage include when the mesh is imbedded and the dissection of the anterior vagina and bladder is extensive.
- Physical restriction after mesh removal surgery is similar to other types of urogynecologic vaginal procedures. Pelvic rest and avoidance of intravaginal intercourse for 6–8 weeks to allow complete healing of the vaginal incisions. Limitations on lifting and straining should be implemented in the immediate postoperative period.

OUTCOMES

- Data regarding outcomes following mesh removal are still emerging.
- Approximately 80% of patients referred to academic centers for mesh removal are reported to have failed medical management, and 15% failed prior partial excisions.
- Reported symptom improvement after mesh graft removal ranges from 25% to 90%, with long-term symptom improvement in approximately 75%.

COMPLICATIONS

- Complications are generally similar to those of mesh placement. The main consideration of limitations is the ability to completely resolve symptoms of pain and to restore pain-free vaginal function.

- Overall risks of intra- or postoperative complications range from 1% to 15%.
  - Infection, bleeding or hematoma, pain: 0% to 10%
  - Bladder or ureteral injury: 1%
  - Exposure: 5% to 19%
  - De novo dyspareunia: 9% to 28%
- Hospital stay, operative time, and need for urologic co-surgeon are all increased with complete excision procedures compared to partial excisions.
- Repeat procedure most often for bothersome recurrent SUI or POP: 20% to 40%.

SUGGESTED READINGS

American Urogynecologic Society and Society of Urodynamics FPMaUR. Position statement on mesh midurethral slings for stress urinary incontinence. 2014. PMID: 24763151 DOI: 10.1097/SPV.0000000000000097

Committee on Gynecologic Practice. Committee opinion no. 513: vaginal placement of synthetic mesh for pelvic organ prolapse. *Obstet Gynecol.* 2011;118(6):1459–1464.

Haylen BT, Freeman RM, Swift SE, et al. An International Urogynecological Association (IUGA)/International Continence Society (ICS) joint terminology and classification of the complications related directly to the insertion of prostheses (meshes, implants, tapes) & grafts in female pelvic floor surgery. *Int Urogynecol J.* 2011;22(1):3–15.

Laycock J. Clinical evaluation of the pelvic floor. In: Schussler B, Laycock J, Norton P, Stanton SL, eds. *Pelvic Floor Re-Education*. London, United Kingdom: Springer-Verlag; 1994:42–48.

Ridgeway B, Walters MD, Paraiso MF, et al. Early experience with mesh excision for adverse outcomes after transvaginal mesh placement using prolapse kits. *Am J Obstet Gynecol.* 2008;199(6):703, e1–e7.

Rogo-Gupta L, Huynh L, Hartshorn TG, Rodriguez LV, Raz S. Long-term symptom improvement and overall satisfaction after prolapse and incontinence graft removal. *Female Pelvic Med Reconstr Surg.* 2013;19(6):352–355.

Tijdink MM, Vierhout ME, Heesakkers JP, Withagen MI. Surgical management of mesh-related complications after prior pelvic floor reconstructive surgery with mesh. *Int Urogynecol J.* 2011;22(11):1395–1404.

Chapter 9
Urethral Diverticulum and Anterior Vaginal Wall Cysts

Christopher M. Tarnay, Morgan E. Fullerton

GENERAL PRINCIPLES
IMAGING AND OTHER DIAGNOSTICS
PREOPERATIVE PLANNING
SURGICAL MANAGEMENT
PROCEDURES AND TECHNIQUES
    Transvaginal Urethral Diverticulectomy
    Transurethral Diverticulotomy or Unroofing
    Skene Gland Cyst Excision
    Anterior Vaginal Wall Cyst Excision
PEARLS AND PITFALLS
POSTOPERATIVE CARE
OUTCOMES
COMPLICATIONS

Urethral Diverticulum and Anterior Vaginal Wall Cysts

Christopher M. Tarnay, Morgan E. Fullerton

GENERAL PRINCIPLES

Definition

- Urethral diverticula are outpouchings of the urethra. Generally, they are thought to form in response to an infection that causes chronic obstruction of the periurethral glands. Over time the chronic obstruction leads to the buildup of secretion which leads to dilation of the glands and an inflammation leads to fibrosis of the glandular wall. Urethral diverticula can also arise as an inflammatory response to urethral surgery or traumatic vaginal delivery. The incidence of urethral diverticula is 6 to 20 per 1,000,000 women, and they account for 1.4% of cases of urinary incontinence in women. Over half of urethral diverticula can be palpated as a cystic mass along the anterior vaginal wall; they represent approximately 80% of periurethral masses. On exam, they are usually tender to palpation and often can be "milked" with subsequent expression of urine or purulent material from the urethral meatus (Fig. 9.1). Rarely, a firm mass is appreciated and this can indicate a stone within the diverticular cavity or suggest the rare finding of malignancy. They can vary in size and can be multiple. The urethral diverticulum is "circumferential" if the outpouching grows to encase the urethra and is "saddlebag" when most of the urethra is surrounded (Fig. 9.2). Patients will usually present with a triad of symptoms that have been referred to as the three Ds—dyspareunia, dysuria, and post-void dribbling. Other common presenting symptoms include urinary incontinence, urinary frequency and urgency, abnormal discharge, and recurrent urinary tract infections (UTI).
- Skene gland cysts are cysts of the paraurethral glands. Skene glands are the female homologue of the prostate glands. Like urethral diverticula, they are usually a result of an infection causing obstruction of the gland opening leading to dilation and inflammation. They present as periurethral masses that can be tender on exam and produce discharge upon milking, but unlike urethral diverticulum, the discharge will come from the

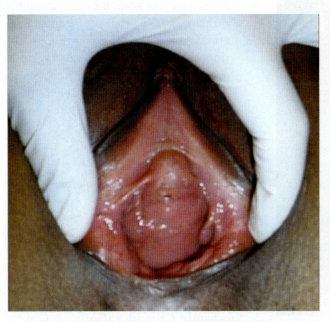
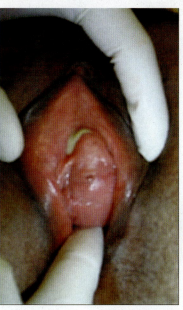

Figure 9.1. **A:** Urethral diverticulum presenting as a large midline periurethral mass. **B:** When palpated or milked, the urethral diverticulum can produce purulent material from the urethral meatus.

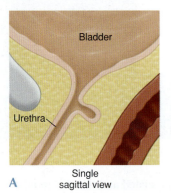 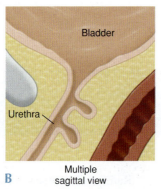 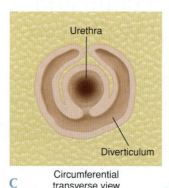 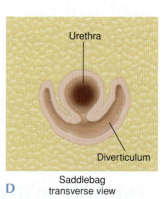

Figure 9.2. Urethral diverticula can be single, multiple, circumferential, or saddlebag. **A:** Sagittal view of single diverticulum. **B:** Sagittal view of multiple diverticula. **C:** Transverse view of circumferential diverticulum. **D:** Transverse view of saddlebag diverticulum.

gland opening which is lateral to the urethra (Fig. 9.3). Symptoms include dyspareunia, dysuria, UTIs, and obstructive voiding symptoms.

- Müllerian duct cysts are the most common cysts of embryologic origin in the anterior vaginal wall. They are remnants of the paramesonephric ducts that give rise to the uterus, cervix, and upper two-thirds of the vagina. Size can be variable from subcentimeter to multiple centimeters, though typically small and asymptomatic, and usually do not require surgical intervention.

- Gartner duct cysts, also known as Wolffian duct cysts, are masses in the anterior vaginal wall that arise from embryologic remnants like Müllerian duct cysts. They are remnants from the mesonephric ducts that typically regress in females, as they give rise to the male urogenital structures of the epididymis, vas deferens, and seminal vesicles. Similar to Müllerian duct cysts, their size can be variable, and if small and asymptomatic do not necessarily require surgical intervention. It is important to note that the finding of Gartner duct cysts can be associated with renal anomalies including renal agenesis or hypoplasia or ectopic ureter on the ipsilateral side. Imaging on these patients should include an evaluation of the upper urinary tract. Gartner duct cysts can grow to several centimeters and can mimic prolapse.

- Epidermal cysts are made up of squamous epithelium within the vaginal wall. They are termed epidermal inclusion cysts when they are due to buried skin fragments that are a product of vaginal surgery, including episiotomies. Their location is not limited to the anterior vaginal wall. They can vary in size and rarely cause symptoms. Contents typically contain a sebaceous-like material. These cysts only require surgical intervention if symptomatic causing pressure or discomfort.

Differential Diagnosis

- Urethral diverticulum
- Distal anterior vaginal prolapse (cystourethrocele)
- Skene gland cyst
- Müllerian duct cyst
- Gartner duct cyst
- Urethral caruncle
- Epidermal cyst
- Leiomyoma

Anatomic Considerations

- When a mass is appreciated in the anterior vaginal wall, it is important to distinguish its relationship to

Figure 9.3. Skene gland cyst appears similar to a urethral diverticulum as it is a periurethral mass; however, a Skene gland cyst is lateral in location as opposed to midline.

the urethra. Specifically, the only mass that should be in direct communication with the urethra is a urethral diverticulum. Other masses in the anterior vaginal wall may be in close proximity but are not connected. Surgically, it is important to distinguish if the mass is separate or connected to the urethra, so that if the surgeon anticipates entry into the urethra, surgical steps can be performed to prevent the risk of fistula formation.

Nonoperative Management

- For urethral diverticula, conservative management with observation can be considered if patients are asymptomatic. Typically, the patient is presenting with symptoms of dyspareunia, dysuria, and postvoid dribbling, and the most effective and definitive way to manage these symptoms are with surgical excision. If surgical intervention is deferred, patients may benefit from manual decompression of the diverticulum after voiding to prevent dribbling and urinary stasis.
- For cysts of the anterior vaginal wall, including Skene gland cysts, Müllerian duct cysts, Gartner duct cysts, and epidermal cysts; they can be observed until they become symptomatic. When these cysts are small, they are typically incidental findings on exam. Once they reach larger sizes and distort the normal anatomy of the vagina, they can cause symptoms of pelvic pressure and dyspareunia. Skene gland cysts can also become infected as they communicate with vaginal flora. It is in those situations where they become symptomatic with tenderness or pain that surgical excision can be considered.

IMAGING AND OTHER DIAGNOSTICS

- The current standard of imaging for urethral diverticula is magnetic resonance imaging (MRI). This noninvasive and nonradiating modality allows detailed imaging of the soft tissues in the pelvis. MRI should be able to confirm whether the lesion is communicating with the urethra, origin location, size, and number. MRI is best performed with the bladder empty so that the urethral diverticula will be filled with urine and will thereby appear bright white on T2-weighted images (Fig. 9.4). MRI is limited by the cost and access. If MRI is unavailable, alternative imaging may be pursued.
- The most common alternative to MRI for the evaluation of urethral diverticulum is ultrasound (US) (Fig. 9.5). This can be done transvaginally or transperineally. Like most studies with US, the sensitivity of the study is dependent on the technician's experience.
- Both MRI and US can be used to evaluate the other types of anterior vaginal wall cysts and can help characterize their location and origin.
- Other imaging techniques that have been used for the evaluation of urethral diverticula are double-balloon positive-pressure urethrography (PPUG) and video cystourethrography (VCUG) (Fig. 9.6). Both studies are no longer routinely performed due to their use of radiation, their need for special equipment and training to perform, and the availability of MRI and/or US. PPUG uses fluoroscopy to take images of the urethral diverticulum, as contrast is instilled into the urethra via a double-balloon catheter. The balloons on the catheter obstruct the proximal and distal ends of the urethra so that the

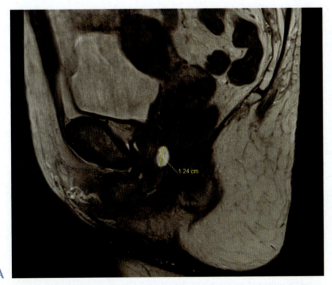
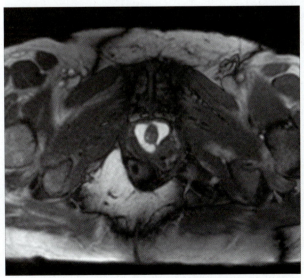

Figure 9.4. MRI of urethral diverticulum. **A:** MRI, T2-weighted midline sagittal view of urethral diverticulum. Appears bright on T2-weighted images. **B:** The diverticulum appears bright and almost completely surrounds the urethra and is considered circumferential or horseshoe.

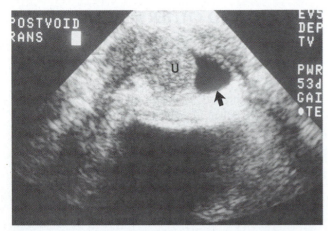

Figure 9.5. Ultrasound coronal view image of urethral diverticulum, cystic-appearing mass near the urethra. U, urethra. (From Dunnick NR, Newhouse JH, Cohan RH, Maturen KE. *Genitourinary Radiology*. 6th ed. Philadelphia, PA: Wolters Kluwer; 2017.)

pressure gradient causes the contrast to fill the diverticula. VCUG also uses fluoroscopy, but it is done while the patient is voiding contrast material that has been instilled into the bladder. The contrast should fill the diverticular cavity while voiding, but it can be inconsistent.

PREOPERATIVE PLANNING

- Evaluation for infection is important in preparing for surgery, especially if the patient has a history of recurrent UTIs. This evaluation includes a urine analysis, urine culture, and if possible, a culture of the diverticular secretions obtained on physical exam. This provides the opportunity for appropriate treatment of any infection prior to surgery.
- Cystourethroscopy can also help with preoperative planning. The objective of the cystourethroscopy is to identify the diverticular ostia number and location. Typically, the ostia are located on the posterior surface of the distal two-thirds of the urethra.
- Urodynamic studies may also be performed if the patient's presenting symptoms include urinary incontinence, and there is concern for stress urinary incontinence (SUI).
- As many as half of the patients who have a urethral diverticulum will have SUI. The patient should be counseled on their options for concomitant procedure in the operating room with urethral diverticulectomy versus a staged procedure with management of SUI after urethral diverticulum management if their symptoms are persistent and bothersome. The 2010 Update of American Urologic Association (AUA) Guideline on the Surgical Management of Female Stress Urinary Incontinence states that despite a paucity of peer-reviewed literature on the subject, it is not advised to use synthetic mesh for the treatment of SUI in the setting of urethral diverticulum due to the presumed increased risk of mesh complications of exposure, erosion into the urethra, infection, or granuloma formation. If a concomitant procedure is planned, an autologous fascial sling or biologic alternative should be used. There are minimal published data on the use of tension-free vaginal tape (TVT) at the time of urethral diverticulectomy with no complications reported. This limited data is insufficient to support the use of synthetic mesh at this time. The benefits of a concomitant procedure are that it saves the patient an additional trip to the operating room with additional anesthesia exposure and recovery time and they have sooner resolution of their SUI symptoms. The benefit of a staged procedure is that up to 80% of patients may no longer have bothersome symptoms after removal of the urethral diverticulum and they can avoid potentially unnecessary surgical risks.

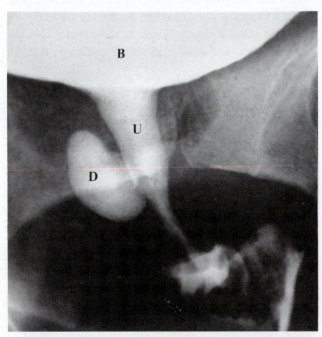

Figure 9.6. Fluoroscopic image of a urethral diverticulum from voiding cystourethrography. B, bladder; U, urethra; D, urethral diverticulum. (From Brant WE, Helms CA. *Brant and Helms Solution*. Philadelphia, PA: Wolters Kluwer; 2006.)

SURGICAL MANAGEMENT

- The goal of surgery is to excise the urethral diverticulum or anterior vaginal wall cyst in its entirety to resolve symptoms and reduce the risk of recurrence.
- Surgical management should be postponed in the setting of active infection as there is increased risk of complications. Treatment with antibiotics or incision

and drainage as needed to be followed by excision and repair at a later date is recommended.
- Surgical intervention for anterior vaginal wall cysts is indicated when they are large and symptomatic. If they are small and asymptomatic, surgical excision is not necessary.

Positioning

- The approach to excision of urethral diverticulum or an anterior vaginal wall cyst is almost universally transvaginal. To obtain adequate access and visualization, the patient should be in dorsal lithotomy.
- Trendelenburg positioning facilitates access to the anterior vaginal wall.
- The arms may be out to facilitate the anesthesia team's access for peripheral lines and monitoring as needed.
- Of note, alternate descriptions of the procedure have the patient in a prone position or Sims position.

Approach

- For urethral diverticulum the most common approach is transvaginal surgical excision. Though, endoscopic approach or marsupialization can be considered.
- For anterior vaginal wall cysts, transvaginal excision is also recommended. Marsupialization can be considered for Skene gland cysts, but there is no mandate to preserve the gland.

Transvaginal Urethral Diverticulectomy

- The patient should be placed in dorsal lithotomy position.
- Prophylactic antibiotics should be administered, typically a first-generation cephalosporin.
- Cystourethroscopy should be performed to identify and localize the location and number of ostia of the urethral diverticula.
- A 14- to 18-French Foley catheter is then placed for drainage of the bladder and to clearly identify the urethra and bladder neck (Tech Fig. 9.1).

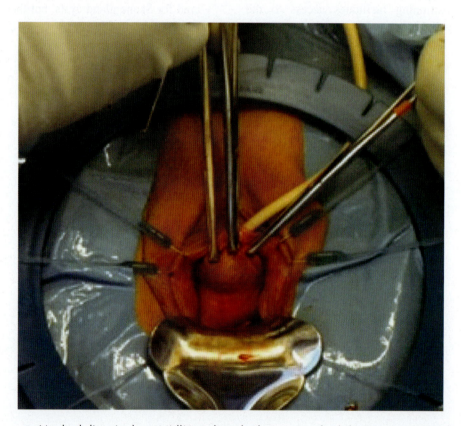

Tech Figure 9.1. Urethral diverticulum. Midline suburethral mass. Urethral diverticulum identified.

- Local anesthesia with vasoconstrictors may be injected at the site of the surgery to reduce blood loss, assist with local pain control, and aid with hydrodissection.
- An inverted-U incision is then made through the vaginal mucosa on the anterior wall along the length of the urethra encompassing the urethral diverticulum.
- A vaginal epithelial flap is further developed with sharp and blunt dissection proximally to the level of the bladder neck and laterally out to the ischiopubic rami.
- The periurethral fascia lying between the anterior vaginal wall and urethral diverticulum should be dissected off the urethral diverticulum using sharp and blunt dissection.
- The incision of the periurethral fascia should be made in a transverse fashion and as much tissue as possible should be preserved to assist with closure (Tech Fig. 9.2).
- After repair of the urethra the periurethral fascia should be identified and closed over defect. This is critical to promote healing and provide support to reduce risk of SUI.

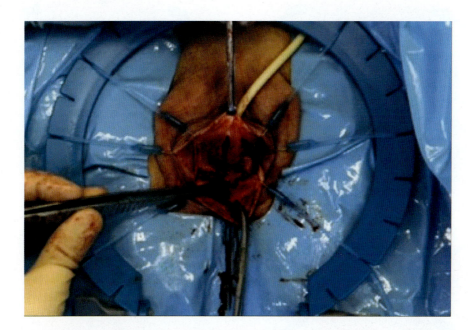

Tech Figure 9.2. Incision into diverticulum. Urethral diverticular sac being dissected from the urethra.

- The diverticulum should then be clearly identified and removed at its base where it connects to the urethra (Tech Fig. 9.3). Caution should be made to avoid enlarging the neck and defect.

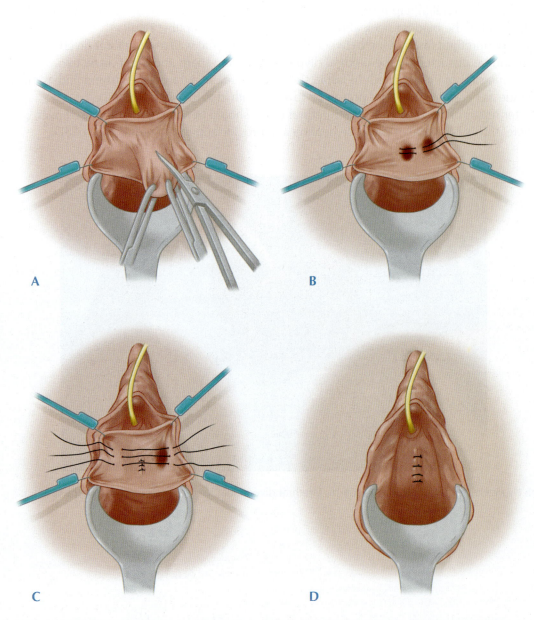

Tech Figure 9.3. Schematic of a series of steps for urethral diverticulectomy. A: Dissection of urethral diverticulum. B: Closure of urethral opening after diverticulum is transected. C: Closure of periurethral fascia. D: Closure of vaginal epithelium.

- The subsequent defect in the urethra is then repaired with 3.0 absorbable suture over the Foley catheter. Care must be taken to ensure the repair is not on tension; therefore, a smaller-caliber catheter is suggested. Ensure no inclusion of the catheter itself by sliding the catheter intermittently.
- If the defect is large and cannot be repaired in a tension-free manner, then reconstruction can be performed with portions of the diverticulum itself or flaps mobilized from the vagina or labia.
- If there are multiple diverticula, the procedure is repeated for each one.
- If it is a circumferential or saddlebag type diverticulum and unable to be easily dissected, the affected portion of the urethra may need to be completely excised and reconstructed with an end-to-end anastomosis.
- The Foley catheter can then be partially removed and fluid instilled into the urethra to ensure the incision is watertight.
- The periurethral fascia is then closed attempts to ensure there is minimal overlapping of the suture line with the urethral repair.
- If there is a large defect, minimal periurethral fascia, or poor tissue quality, then a Martius flap may be additionally performed to assist in healing.
- If the patient had SUI prior to the procedure and a decision had been made to proceed with a concomitant sling, it would be placed at this time. Given the urethra is entered during the diverticulectomy, an autologous fascial sling or biologic alternative is preferred.
- The vaginal epithelial flap is then reapproximated with absorbable suture and hemostasis is confirmed.
- To protect the urethral repair and drain the bladder, the indwelling foley catheter should remain 7 to 21 days.
- If a suprapubic catheter was placed for drainage of the bladder, a Foley catheter is still left in place but can be capped.

Transurethral Diverticulotomy or Unroofing

- This procedure was first described in the literature in 1979 by Dr. Jack Lapides with the objective to extend the ostium of the urethral diverticulum to allow for full communication of the diverticular cavity with the urethra.
- The patient should be placed in dorsal lithotomy.
- A rigid resectoscope is used to visualize the ostium of the urethral diverticulum, the resectoscope is then angled to be parallel with the lumen of the urethra, and a curved knife electrode is then introduced into the ostium (Tech Fig. 9.4).
- The resectoscope is then straightened and elevated so that the knife electrode is tenting up the urethral diverticular cavity toward the posterior urethral wall.
- The knife electrode is then advanced on cutting or blended current to divide the entire roof of the diverticular cavity. Ultimately, this incision may extend along most of the length of the urethra.
- A Foley catheter is placed and maintained overnight.

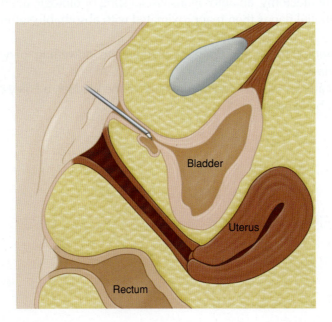

Tech Figure 9.4. Transurethral diverticulotomy. Cystoscope with knife electrode is used to enlarge the diverticular opening in the urethra.

Skene Gland Cyst Excision

- The patient should be placed in dorsal lithotomy.
- Cystourethroscopy is performed to confirm the diagnosis of Skene gland cyst and that there is no communication with the urethra. A Foley catheter should then be placed.
- A similar inverted-U incision, as described for urethral diverticulectomy, may be performed.
- Alternately, an vertical incision may be made over the vaginal bulge extending superior end at the opening of the Skene gland (Tech Fig. 9.5).

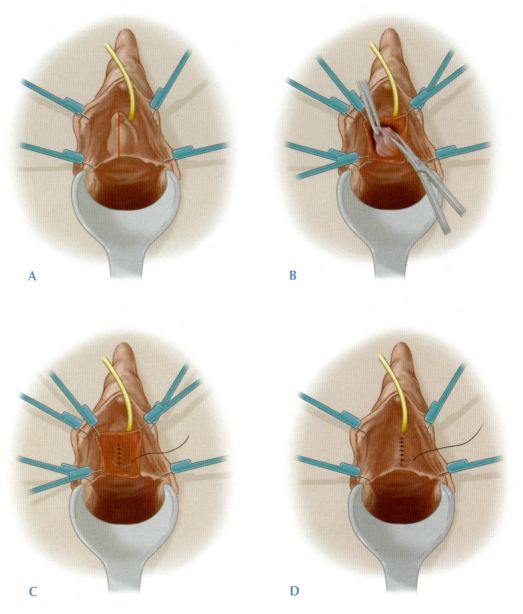

Tech Figure 9.5. Schematic of Skene gland cyst excision. **A:** Identification of Skene gland cyst. Incision over area of maximal distension. **B:** Dissection of Skene gland cyst from vaginal epithelium. **C:** Closure of defect left by Skene gland cyst removal with absorbable suture. **D:** Closure of vaginal epithelium with absorbable suture.

- The cyst may then be dissected out using sharp and blunt dissection until completely identified. Attempts are made to remove the cyst intact, but rupture is common. If cyst rupture occurs, attempts should be made to completely dissect out the entire cyst cavity.
- The resulting defect left by the removal of the cyst should be reapproximated with absorbable suture.
- The overlying vaginal epithelium is then reapproximated with absorbable suture.
- Foley catheter may be used for 3 to 5 days after surgery.

Anterior Vaginal Wall Cyst Excision

- The approach to surgical removal of anterior vaginal wall cysts are similar to a Skenes gland excision. Gartners duct cysts can be very deep and addressing the dead space with layered closure is important.
- The patient should be placed in dorsal lithotomy and stirrups with antibiotic and venous thromboembolism prophylaxis as previously described.
- The anterior vaginal wall cyst is identified and an incision is made with a scalpel over the most prominent bulge of the cyst, typically in a longitudinal fashion.
- The cyst is then dissected out using sharp and blunt dissection until completely identified. Attempts are made to remove the cyst intact, but rupture is common. If the cyst is ruptured, attempts should be made to completely dissect out the entire cyst cavity.
- The resulting defect left by the removal of the cyst should be reapproximated with absorbable suture. If deep, then layered closure should be performed.
- The overlying vaginal epithelium is then reapproximated with absorbable suture.
- Vaginal packing can be considered.

PEARLS AND PITFALLS

CYSTOURETHROSCOPY

- Should be performed at the start of surgery. In the setting of urethral diverticula, it can assist with determining location and number, and in the setting of a presumed Skene gland cyst, it can confirm that it is not communicating with the urethra.

TENSION-FREE CLOSURE

- Care should be taken to ensure the closure of the urethra is tension free to reduce the risk of breakdown of the repair.

AVOID OVERLAPPING SUTURE LINES

- Care should be taken to avoid overlapping suture lines in the closure to reduce the risk of urethrovaginal fistula formation. For this reason, an inverted-U incision is made in the vaginal mucosa and the periurethral fascial incision should be made in a transverse fashion.

CONCOMITANT MANAGEMENT OF SUI

- If a patient has SUI preoperatively, the option of a concomitant procedure versus staged procedure should be discussed with the patient. If the patient desires a concomitant procedure, should proceed with an autologous fascial sling or biologic alternative, as a mesh sling has a presumed increased risk of erosion and wound breakdown.

MARTIUS FLAP

- When there is minimal periurethral fascia to close between the urethra and vaginal mucosa or there is a large urethral defect, a Martius flap should be considered to assist in the integrity of the repair and reduce risk of wound breakdown and urethrovaginal fistula formation.

POSTOPERATIVE CARE

- After diverticulectomy, a 14- to 18-French Foley catheter is maintained for 7 to 21 days depending on the extent of surgical manipulation. Imaging can be considered prior to removal of the Foley catheter to confirm urethral integrity. Anticholinergics can be offered to prevent bladder spasms while the Foley catheter is in place based on provider preference.
- Antibiotics are commonly extended postoperatively after urethral diverticulectomy. Typically, IV antibiotics are administered overnight if the patient is admitted for observation and then a course of oral antibiotics is continued while the Foley catheter is in place. In one review of urethral diverticulum management by Crescenze and Goldman published in 2015, they note that there are no data to suggest improved outcomes with extended antibiotics past the initial preoperative prophylaxis if the workup for infection is negative, though they still prescribe them.
- If vaginal packing was placed it should be removed prior to discharge and within 48 hours of surgery.
- In the setting of Skene gland cyst excision, a Foley catheter is also left in place for 3 to 5 days. Antibiotics and anticholinergics can be considered for the duration of the catheter.
- With other vaginal cyst removals, urinary catheters and antibiotics are not routine.
- Pain control with oral analgesics as necessary.
- Early ambulation and resumption of normal daily activities can resume soon after surgery. Pelvic rest should be observed for at least 6 weeks.

OUTCOMES

- The cure rate of urethral diverticulectomy ranges from 70% to 90%. Recurrence of urethral diverticula is more common in cases where there were multiple diverticula, the diverticula were more proximal or circumferential, or if the patient had undergone previous repairs.

- For vaginal cyst excisions, specifically Skene gland cyst excision, there are limited data on outcomes, but in the reported literature, the recurrence rate is low at 0% to 6%.

COMPLICATIONS

- Common early postoperative complications are urinary retention and infection.
- The most devastating complication is urethrovaginal fistula formation. This is a late complication and occurs in up to 6% of cases. Patients will usually report involuntary and persistent leakage of urine. This sequelae requires additional surgery to repair after the initial diverticulectomy has healed. The principles employed during urethral diverticulectomy to avoid fistula formation are a tension-free closure, avoidance of overlapping suture lines, and mobilization of vascular tissue as needed, usually with a Martius flap.
- De novo SUI can present in up to one-third of patients, which may require subsequent surgical intervention. This is presumed to be due to disruption of the urethral support.
- Other less commonly reported complications include de novo urinary urgency incontinence and urethral stricture.
- Persistent or new onset of chronic pain is always a risk after any surgery. With vaginal procedures, there is also the concern of new-onset dyspareunia from scar tissue.

SUGGESTED READINGS

Aspera AM, Rackley RR, Vasavada SP. Contemporary evaluation and management of the female urethral diverticulum. *Urol Clin North Am.* 2002;29:617–624.

Bodner-Adler B, Halpern K, Hanzal E. Surgical management of urethral diverticula in women: a systematic review. *Int Urogynecol J.* 2016;27:993–1001.

Crescenze IM, Goldman HB. Female urethral diverticulum: current diagnosis and management. *Curr Urol Rep.* 2015;16:71.

Dmochowski RR, Blaivas JM, Gormley EA, et al. Update of AUA guideline on the surgical management of female stress urinary incontinence. *J Urol.* 2010;183:1906–1914.

Eilber KS, Raz S. Benign cystic lesions of the vagina: a literature review. *J Urol.* 2003;170:717–722.

El-Nashar SA, Bacon MM, Kim-Fine S, Weaver AL, Gebhart JB, Klingele CJ. Incidence of female urethral diverticulum: a population-based analysis and literature review. *Int Urogynecol J.* 2014;25:73–79.

Foster J, Lemack G, Zimmern P. Skene's gland cyst excision. *Int Urogynecol J.* 2016;27:817–820.

Ko KJ, Suh YS, Kim TH, et al. Surgical outcomes of primary and recurrent female urethral diverticula. *Urology.* 2017;105:181–185.

Lapides J. Transurethral treatment of urethral diverticula in women. *J Urol.* 1979;121:736–738.

Reeves FA, Inman RD, Chapple CR. Management of symptomatic urethral diverticula in women: a single-centre experience. *Eur Urol.* 2014;66:164–172.

Spence HM, Duckett JW, Jr. Diverticulum of the female urethra: clinical aspects and presentation of a simple operative technique for cure. *J Urol.* 1970;104:432–437.

Chapter 10
Cystoscopy
Lisa Rogo-Gupta

GENERAL PRINCIPLES
PREOPERATIVE PLANNING
SURGICAL MANAGEMENT
PROCEDURES AND TECHNIQUES
    Endoscope Insertion
    Bladder Evaluation
    Ureteral Patency
PEARLS AND PITFALLS
POSTOPERATIVE CARE
OUTCOMES
COMPLICATIONS

Cystoscopy

Lisa Rogo-Gupta

GENERAL PRINCIPLES

Definition

- **Cystoscopy** is a procedure wherein the lower urinary tract is visualized endoscopically. Entry is through the urethra and also allows visualization of the urethral lumen. Often cystoscopy is referred to as *cystourethroscopy*.
  - **Diagnostic cystoscopy** is performed for the purpose of evaluation and diagnosis. This procedure is minimally invasive and causes only mild discomfort and can often be performed in the office setting under local anesthesia alone.
    - It is routinely done in conjunction with urogynecologic procedures.
  - **Operative cystoscopy** is performed for the purpose of accomplishing a surgical objective. This procedure is minimally invasive but may cause moderate discomfort, require operative instruments or energy-based treatment, and is often performed under additional anesthesia.

PREOPERATIVE PLANNING

- Indications for preoperative **diagnostic cystoscopy** in urogynecology
  - Evaluation of lower urinary tract pathology.
    - Lower urinary tract symptoms (LUTS)
    - Overactive bladder (OAB); severe
      - Routine cystoscopy is **not indicated** in the routine evaluation of *uncomplicated* stress urinary incontinence or mild OAB. Risk of associated malignancy is low in such cases at approximately 2%.[1]
      - Cystoscopy **should be considered** in patients who fail first-line therapies prior to performance of reversible or invasive interventions.[2]
    - Interstitial cystitis/painful bladder syndrome (IC/PBS)[3]
    - Hematuria[4]
    - Recurrent urinary tract infections
    - Urethral diverticulum
    - Urethral stricture
    - Urinary tract fistula
    - Previous mesh surgery
- Indications for diagnostic cystoscopy during surgery
  - Routine following surgical procedures whose risks include injury to the lower urinary tract.
  - Risk of lower urinary tract injury ranges from 0.01% to 0.08% during hysterectomy and gynecologic procedures performed for benign disease.[5]
    - Hysterectomy (vaginal, abdominal, laparoscopic)
    - Pelvic organ prolapse repair (cystocele, enterocele, vault suspension, colpocleisis)
    - Urinary incontinence procedures (sling, Burch, bladder neck suspension), as these procedures carry a 3% to 9% overall risk of perforation
    - Lysis of adhesions (endometriosis, malignancy, adnexal pathology)
- Indications for **operative cystoscopy** in urogynecology
  - Procedures performed on the lower urinary tract
    - Urinary incontinence procedures (urethral bulking injection, injection of botulinum toxin)
    - Bladder hydrodistension
    - Fulguration of ulceration
    - Foreign body removal (stone, prosthetic implant, suture material)
    - Lesion biopsy
    - Transurethral incision of the bladder neck
    - Ureteral stent insertion
    - Suprapubic catheter insertion
    - Urethral diverticulum excision
    - Urethroplasty
    - Fistula repair
- Urinary tract infection should not be present at the time of routine cystoscopy. Routine antibiotics are not recommended for the majority of cystoscopic procedures.[6,7]
  - Consideration for antibiotics include:
    - Active infection
    - Immunosuppression
    - Bacterial colonization (indwelling catheter, fistula)
    - Population-based risks (cost, microbial resistance)

SURGICAL MANAGEMENT

Positioning

- Cystoscopy is performed with the patient in lithotomy position similar to other gynecologic procedures (Fig. 10.1).
  - Various lithotomy stirrups are available to assure patient safety and comfort, minimizing risk for related injury.

Approach

- Although cystoscopy is considered a clean-contaminated procedure, most facilities ensure that all equipment is sterile to prevent cross contamination. Cystoscopy is performed either in the office or operating room setting which should be selected based on the procedural indication, anticipated findings, and consideration of patient comfort.
- Diagnostic and operative cystoscopy can both often be performed using minimal anesthesia. Lidocaine can be inserted into the urethra and bladder in viscous or gel form without the use of needle puncture. Additional anesthetic approaches such as sedation, regional or general, can be used when additional discomfort is anticipated.
- Distending fluid is utilized for visualization. Saline or sterile water may be used for diagnostic cystoscopy, however when using electrocautery, a nonconducting solution such as glycine or sterile water is required.
- Appropriate instruments should be prepared prior to the procedure.
  - Cystoscopy can be performed using a flexible or rigid instrument.
    - Rigid instruments are typically used on female patients and are approximately 30 cm in length.
    - Operative tools are available such as forceps, resectoscope, lasers, coagulation electrodes, stone baskets, and stents.
- Optimal lens angle should also be considered. The 0- or 12-degree lenses are ideal for evaluating the urethral lumen or performing cystoscopic injections. The 30- and 70-degree lenses are often best used for diagnostic cystoscopy requiring visualization of ureters, base of the bladder, and the trigone.
- One example is bladder perforation of mid-urethral slings, which is often located close to the bladder neck (Fig. 10.2).

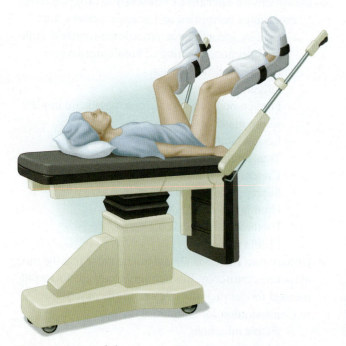

Figure 10.1. Low lithotomy position for cystoscopy.

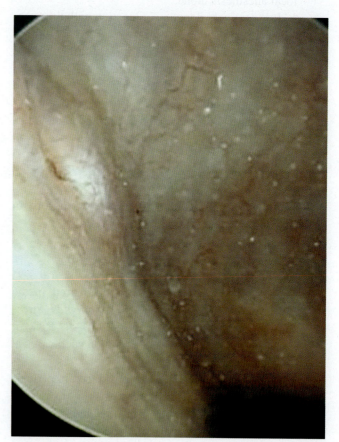

Figure 10.2. Cystoscopic view of ureteral opening.

Endoscope Insertion

- The endoscope is inserted through the urethral meatus into the bladder.
- The urethral meatus and lumen should be inspected during insertion and any relevant findings documented.

Instrumentation for Cystoscopy

- Cystoscopic evaluation of urethra and bladder **(Video 10.1)**.

Bladder Evaluation

- The bladder is systematically evaluated. Orientation can be achieved by inserting cystoscope into the bladder and withdrawing to the internal urethral meatus (bladder neck). Typically, inspection begins at the dome of the bladder with an often-seen small air bubble representing the most superior aspect of the bladder. The cystoscope is then manipulated such that the bladder wall can be inspected completely, including the trigone, the interureteric ridge, and ureteral orifices. Common approaches include inspection by quadrants, circular rings, or spokes (Tech Fig. 10.1).

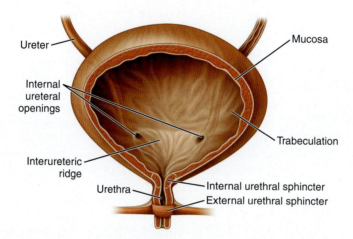

Tech Figure 10.1. Bladder anatomy. (Modified from Archer P, Nelson LA. *Applied Anatomy & Physiology for Manual Therapists*. Philadelphia, PA: Wolters Kluwer; 2012.)

Ureteral Patency

- Ureteral patency is evaluated by visualization of active urine flow into the bladder. This can be performed with or without the use of intravenous solutions or oral phenazopyridine that result in discoloration of the urine to improve visualization of urine jets (see Table 10.1).
- If ureteral patency is not confirmed, next-line options would include ureteral catheter or stent placement and evaluation for location of potential obstruction or injury.

Table 10.1 Medications Used for the Cystoscopic Evaluation of Ureteral Patency

Medication	Dosage Details	Metabolism	Consideration(s)
Phenazopyridine (analgesic)	• 200 mg PO 0.5–5 hours prior to cystoscopy • PO half-life 7 hours	• Renal and hepatic	• Contraindications: G6PD deficiency
Methylene blue (monoamine oxidase inhibitor)	• 50 mg IV over 5 minutes • 10 mL vial, 10 mg/mL • IV half-life 5–6.5 hours	• Renal • 75% metabolized to colorless leucomethylene blue	• Not FDA approved • Can cause methemoglobinemia at high doses (>7 mg/kg) • Can cause serotonin syndrome in patients taking serotonergic agents • Contraindications: renal impairment, G6PD deficiency, pediatric patients
Sodium fluorescein	• 5 mL 10% vial • Use 0.2–0.5 mL IV • IV half-life 4–5 hours	• Renal	• Not FDA approved • Can stain skin and sclera yellow in high doses
Indigo carmine (pH indicator, FD&C Blue #2)	• 50 mL IV • 5 mL vial, 8 mg/mL • IV half-life 4–5 minutes • Given 10–15 minutes prior to cystoscopy	• Renal	• Not FDA approved • Short supply in US • No known drug interactions

PEARLS AND PITFALLS

PREOPERATIVE PAIN ASSESSMENT

- Performing preoperative pain assessment that includes anticipated procedural details, patient pain threshold, and pain control requirements will assist in appropriate scheduling and setting patient expectations, increasing the likelihood of a successful procedure.

ANTICIPATE INSTRUMENT NEEDS

- Having multiple lens angle options and operative tools available for the procedure will increase the likelihood of a successful procedure.

USE CAUTION DURING CYSTOSCOPE INSERTION

- Inserting the cystoscope into the urethra and bladder under direct visualization and at a cautious pace will decrease the risk of complications such as perforation.

POSTOPERATIVE CARE

- Postoperative care following urogynecologic procedures is similar to that for other benign gynecologic surgeries.

OUTCOMES

- Outcomes of cystoscopy depend on the findings and procedure performed.

COMPLICATIONS

- Cystoscopy is considered minimally invasive and low risk similar to other urogynecologic procedures.
- Most common complications include mild discomfort or pain, urinary tract infection, and rarely perforation.
- Missed diagnoses are not uncommon among both gynecologists and urologists.[1] Delayed presentation of urinary tract injuries also occur and would not be identified at the time of procedure such as partial ureteral obstruction or particularly with thermal injuries to the lower urinary tract.

KEY REFERENCES

1. Davis R, Jones JS, Barocas DA, et al. Diagnosis, evaluation, and follow-up of asymptomatic microhematuria (AMH) in adults: AUA guideline. *J Urol*. 2012;188(6 Suppl):2473–2481.
2. American College of Obstetricians and Gynecologists. ACOG Committee Opinion. Number 372. July 2007. The role of cystourethroscopy in the generalist obstetrician-gynecologist practice. *Obstet Gynecol*. 2007;110(1):221–224.
3. Committee Opinion No. 603: evaluation of uncomplicated stress urinary incontinence in women before surgical treatment. *Obstet Gynecol*. 2014;123(6):1403–1407.
4. Gormley EA, Lightner DJ, Faraday M, Vasavada SP. Diagnosis and treatment of overactive bladder (non-neurogenic) in adults: AUA/SUFU guideline amendment. *J Urol*. 2015;193(5):1572–1580.
5. Hanno PM, Burks DA, Clemens JQ, et al. AUA guideline for the diagnosis and treatment of interstitial cystitis/bladder pain syndrome. *J Urol*. 2011;185(6):2162–2170.
6. ACOG Committee on Practice Bulletins–Gynecology. ACOG practice bulletin No. 104: antibiotic prophylaxis for gynecologic procedures. *Obstet Gynecol*. 2009;113(5):1180–1189.
7. Wolf JS, Jr, Bennett CJ, Dmochowski RR, et al. Best practice policy statement on urologic surgery antimicrobial prophylaxis. *J Urol*. 2008;179(4):1379–1390.

Index

Note: Page number followed by f, p, and t indicates figure, procedure material, and table, respectively.

A

Abdominal sacrocolpopexy, 54p–55p
Anoscope, 126
Anterior colporrhaphy, 9p–10p
Anterior longitudinal ligament, 52, 52f
Anterior vaginal wall (AVW) prolapse, 3, 3f. *See also* Anterior vaginal wall repair
   differential diagnosis of, 4–5, 5f
   dynamic MRI for, 7, 7f
   hydronephrosis and, 7
   nonoperative management, 5–6, 6f
   symptoms associated with, 3
   urinary symptoms with, evaluation of, 7
Anterior vaginal wall repair
   AVW prolapse and, 3 (*see also* Anterior vaginal wall (AVW) prolapse)
   complications, 15
   diagnostic evaluation, 6–7, 7f
   general principles, 3–6
   history and physical examination, 3–4, 3f, 4t
   indications for, 3
   outcomes, 14–15
   patient positioning, 8
   pearls and pitfalls, 14
   postoperative care, 14
   preoperative planning, 7–8
   procedures and techniques
      graft-augmented repair, 11p
      paravaginal repair, 12p–13p
      traditional midline repair (anterior colporrhaphy), 9p–10p
   surgical management, 8
Apical prolapse repair, abdominal approach, 51–64
   anatomy related to, 51–52, 51f, 52f
   complications, 64
   general principles, 51–52
   outcomes, 63–64
   pearls and pitfalls, 63
   postoperative care, 63
   preoperative planning, 52
   procedures and techniques
      hysteropexy, 62p
      laparoscopic uterosacral ligament suspension, 60p–61p
      robotic-assisted laparoscopic sacrocolpopexy, 56p–59p
   surgical management, 52–53
      approach, 53, 53f
      patient positioning, 53, 53f
Apical prolapse, vaginal repair of
   causes of apical prolapse and, 19, 19f
   complications, 30
   general principles, 19
   imaging studies, 20
   outcomes, 30
   patient positioning, 21
      lithotomy, 21, 21f
   pearls and pitfalls, 30
   postoperative care, 30
   preoperative planning, 20–21
   sacrospinous ligament vault suspension, 26p
      incision and exposure, 26p
      SSL suture attachment to cuff, 28p
      suture placement, 27p
   uterine sparing technique for, 28p
   uterosacral ligament hysteropexy, 29p
      suture attachment to uterus/cervix, 29p
      suture placement, 29p
   uterosacral ligament vault suspension
      positioning and exposure, 22p
      ureteral integrity, 24p
      uterosacral ligament, identification and suture placement, 23p–24p
      vaginal cuff affixation to uterosacral ligament, 25p
   vaginal and pelvic exam, 19–20
   vaginal approach, 21
Arcus tendineus fascia pelvis (ATFP), 12p–13p
AVW prolapse. *See* Anterior vaginal wall (AVW) prolapse

B

Bladder diary, 70, 145
Botulinum toxin, cystoscopic injection of, 71, 86p–87p
Bowel preparation, 20–21

C

Capio suture capturing device, 13p, 27p
Colon transit studies, 36, 36f
Colovaginal fistulas, 125. *See also* Rectovaginal fistulas (RVFs) and perineal lacerations
Colporrhaphy, 143
Computed tomography (CT), for rectovaginal fistulas, 128
Computed tomography urogram, 101
Cystoscopic injection of botulinum toxin, 71
   complications, 96
   outcomes, 95
   procedures and techniques, 86p–87p
Cystoscopy, 175–180
   complications, 180
   diagnostic, 175
   indications for, 175
   operative, 175
   outcomes, 180
   pearls and pitfalls, 180
   postoperative care, 180
   preoperative planning, 175
   procedures and techniques
      bladder evaluation, 178p
      endoscope insertion, 177p
      ureteral patency, 179p
   surgical management
      approach, 176, 176f
      positioning, 176, 176f
Cystourethroscopy, 101, 101f, 160. *See also* Cystoscopy

D

Darifenacin, in urinary incontinence, 69t
Defecograms, 36
DIAPER (mnemonic), 67
Digital rectovaginal exam, 126
Donut pessary, for prolapse, 19, 20f

E

EAS. *See* External anal sphincter (EAS)
Endoanal ultrasound, 36, 37f, 128
Enterocele, 33, 33f
Epidermal cysts, 158. *See also* Urethral diverticulum and anterior vaginal wall cysts
External anal sphincter (EAS), 126, 127f, 129

F

Fecal incontinence, 36
Fesoterodine, in urinary incontinence, 69t
Fistula-in-ano, 125, 125f. *See also* Rectovaginal fistulas (RVFs) and perineal lacerations
Fistulography, 128
Frequency–volume chart, 70, 145

G

Gartner duct cysts, 158. *See also* Urethral diverticulum and anterior vaginal wall cysts

Gellhorn pessary, 6
Genitourinary (GU) fistula
  complications, 121–122
  definition, 99
  diagnostic evaluation, 101
    computed tomography (CT) urogram, 101
    cystourethroscopy, 101, 101f
    hysterogram/saline sonohysterogram, 101
    voiding cystourethrography (VCUG), 101, 101f, 102f
  differential diagnosis, 100
  laparoscopic and robotic-assisted laparoscopic techniques, 114p
    Martius fat pad graft, 115p–117p
    transvaginal gluteal flap, 118p
    transvaginal labial flap, 118p
    transvaginal omental flap, 118p–119p
    transvaginal peritoneal flap, 117p, 119p
    vascular tissue interposition, 114p
    vesicouterine/vesicocervical fistulae, 114p
  nonoperative management, 101
  outcomes, 121
  pearls and pitfalls, 120
  physical examination, 99–100, 100f
  postoperative care, 120–121
    antibiotics, 120
    anticholinergics, 120
    continuous bladder drainage, 120–121
  preoperative planning, 102
  procedures and techniques
    abdominal approach, 109p–113p
    urethrovaginal fistulae, 108p
    vaginal approach, 104p–107p
    vesicovaginal fistulae, 104p–107p
  surgical management, 102
    approach, 103
    patient positioning, 102–103, 102f
  types of, 99, 99f

H
Hysterogram/saline sonohysterogram, 101
Hysteropexy, 62p

I
IAS. *See* Internal anal sphincter (IAS)
Implantable pulse generator (IPG), 88p
Inclusion cyst, 4, 5f
Internal anal sphincter (IAS), 126, 127f, 129

K
Kegel exercises, 6, 69

L
Laceration, obstetric, repair of, 134p–135p. *See also* Rectovaginal fistulas (RVFs) and perineal lacerations

  first- and second-degree lacerations, 134p
  fourth-degree lacerations, 135p
  third-degree lacerations, 134p
Laparoscopic uterosacral ligament suspension, 60p–61p
Lead-pipe urethra, 67
Lone Star self-retaining vaginal retractor, 39f, 39p

M
Magnetic resonance defecography, 36
Magnetic resonance imaging (MRI)
  for rectovaginal fistulas, 128
  for urethral diverticula, 159, 159f
  for vaginal prolapse, 7, 7f, 19
Martius fat pad graft, 115p–117p, 130, 131f
Mesh, 143. *See also* Vaginal mesh, removal of
Mid-urethral slings (MUS), 70, 70f, 143. *See also* Urinary incontinence (UI)
  complications, 95
  outcomes, 95
  placement of
    retropubic approach, 74p–76p
    transobturator approach, 74p, 76p–77p
  procedures and techniques, 73p–80p
  retropubic sling, 73p
  single incision sling, 73p
  surgical approach, 72
  tensioning of, 78p–80p
    with Babcock, 79p
    with with scissor, 79p
  transobturator sling, 73p
Minimally invasive surgery (MIS) approach, for prolapse, 21
Mirabegron, in urinary incontinence, 69t
Mixed urinary incontinence (MUI), 67. *See also* Urinary incontinence (UI)
Miya Hook, 27p
MRI. *See* Magnetic resonance imaging (MRI)
Müllerian duct cysts, 158. *See also* Urethral diverticulum and anterior vaginal wall cysts
MUS. *See* Mid-urethral slings (MUS)

N
Nocturia, 67
Nonsteroidal anti-inflammatory drugs (NSAIDs), 139

O
Obturator foramen anatomy, 77p
Onabotulinum toxin, 86p
Overactive bladder syndrome, 67
Oxybutynin, in urinary incontinence, 69t

P
Pad weight tests, 70
Pediatric laparotomy sponges, 22p

Pelvic organ prolapse (POP), 3, 143
  anterior vaginal wall prolapse (*see* Anterior vaginal wall (AVW) prolapse)
  apical prolapse, 10, 51 (*see also* Apical prolapse, vaginal repair of)
  definition of, 3
  nonoperative management, 5–6, 19, 20f
  symptoms of, 3
Pelvic organ prolapse quantification (POP-Q), 34
Percutaneous nerve evaluation (PNE), 88p
Perineal lacerations, 125, 132. *See also* Rectovaginal fistulas (RVFs) and perineal lacerations
  acute, 132–133
  chronic, 133
  classification of, 125–126, 126f
  risk factors for, 126
Perineal wound breakdown, 133
  secondary closure of, 136p
Pessary, 6, 19, 35
  for anterior vaginal prolapse, 6f
  doughnut, 20f
  Gellhorn, 35f
  for posterior vaginal prolapse, 35–36, 35f
  ring, 20f
  saddle, 36
  types of, 6f
POP. *See* Pelvic organ prolapse (POP)
Positive-pressure urethrography (PPUG), double-balloon, 159–160
Posterior colporrhaphy
  site-specific, 42p
  traditional, 40p–41p
Posterior tibial nerve stimulation (PTNS), 69, 69f
Posterior vaginal wall prolapse
  definition and subtypes, 33
  differential diagnosis, 35
  nonoperative management, 35–36, 35f
  with other pelvic floor defects, 33, 34f
  physical examination, 34–35, 34f
    neurologic exam, 34
    pelvic organ prolapse quantification (POP-Q), 34
    perineal body assessment, 34
    rectovaginal exam, 35
  risk factors for, 33
  symptoms of, 33
Posterior vaginal wall repair, 33–47
  complications
    bleeding, 46
    constipation, 46
    defecatory dysfunction, 47
    dyspareunia, 47
    gluteal pain, 46
    intraoperative, 46
    postoperative, 46–47
    rectal injury, 46

diagnostic imaging
  colon transit studies, 36, 36f
  defecogram, 36
  endoanal ultrasound, 36, 37f
  magnetic resonance defecography, 36
general principles, 33–36
outcomes, 46
pearls and pitfalls, 45
postoperative care, 45–46
  activity restrictions, 45
  antibiotic prophylaxis, 45
  bowel regimen, 45
  follow-up visit, 46
  pelvic rest, 45
preoperative planning, 37
procedures and techniques
  abdominal approach, 44p
  apical detachment, 43p
  graft augmentation, 43p
  site-specific posterior colporrhaphy, 42p
  traditional colporrhaphy, 40p–41p
  vaginal approach, 39p
surgical management, 38
  approach, 38
  patient positioning, 38, 38f
Post-void residual (PVR), 7, 67, 144
Presacral space, 52, 55p
Proctoscopy, 145
Pubovaginal slings, 70, 70f. *See also* Urinary incontinence (UI)
  from biologic material, 81p
  complications, 95
  outcomes, 95
  procedures and techniques, 81p–84p
    biologic sling, 82p
    passage of sling, 83p
    Pereyra-Raz ligature carrier, 82p
PVR. *See* Post-void residual (PVR)

R
Rectocele, 33, 33f
Rectovaginal fistulas (RVFs) and perineal lacerations, 125–140, 125f
  classification systems, 125
    perineal lacerations, 125–126, 126f
  complications after repair, 140
  definition, 125
  diagnostic evaluation, 128
  differential diagnosis, 126
  general principles, 125–128
  nonoperative management, 127–128, 127f
  outcomes, 139
  pearls and pitfalls, 139
  physical examination, 126, 127f
  postoperative care, 139
  preoperative planning, 128
  procedures and techniques
    acute obstetric laceration repairs, 134p–135p
    chronic perineal laceration repair, 137p–138p
    first- and second-degree lacerations, 134p
    fourth-degree lacerations, 135p
    perineal wound breakdown, secondary closure of, 136p
    third-degree lacerations, 134p
  surgical management, 128
    approach to, 129
    fistula fibrin glue and fistula plugs, 132–133, 132f
    interposition of neovascular flap, 130–132, 131f
    patient positioning, 129
    transanal approach, 132, 132f
    transperineal approach, 129–130
    transvaginal approach without sphincteroplasty, 129, 129f
    transvaginal approach with sphincteroplasty, 129, 130f
Ring pessary, for prolapse, 19, 20f
Robotic-assisted laparoscopic sacrocolpopexy, 56p–59p

S
Sacral neuromodulation, 71, 71f, 94. *See also* Urinary incontinence (UI)
  assessment of results, 93p
  complications, 96
  implantable pulse generator, 88p
  outcomes, 95
  percutaneous evaluation, 92p
  percutaneous implantation, 88p
  procedures and techniques, 88p–93p
  staged implantation
    first stage, 89p–92p
    second stage, 92p
  wound infection, 93p
Sacrohysteropexy, 62p
Sacrospinous ligament vault suspension, for apical prolapse, 26p–27p
Seton stitch, 127, 127f
Sigmoidocele, 33
Silastic Foley catheter, 122
Skene gland cysts, 157–158, 158f. *See also* Urethral diverticulum and anterior vaginal wall cysts
Solifenacin, in urinary incontinence, 69t
Spondylodiscitis, 52
Stress urinary incontinence (SUI), 67, 160. *See also* Urinary incontinence (UI)
Suprapubic catheters, 121
Surgical care improvement project (SCIP), 95

T
Tampon test, 100, 100f
Tension-free vaginal tape (TVT), 160
Tolterodine, in urinary incontinence, 69t
Transurethral bulking, 70–71, 71f. *See also* Urinary incontinence (UI)
  complications, 96
  outcomes, 95
  procedures and techniques, 85p–87p
Trospium, in urinary incontinence, 69t

U
UI. *See* Urinary incontinence (UI)
Ultrasound (US)
  mesh visualization by, 145, 145f
  for rectovaginal fistulas, 128
  for urethral diverticula, 159, 160f
  for vaginal prolapse, 19
Upsylon mesh, 59p
Ureteral efflux visualization, 20
Ureteral kinking, 24p, 30
Ureteral patency, cystoscopic evaluation of, 179p
Ureteral stent placement, 101
Urethral diverticulum and anterior vaginal wall cysts, 157–171
  anatomic considerations, 158–159
  complications, 171
  differential diagnosis, 158
  general principles
    epidermal cysts, 158
    Gartner duct cysts, 158
    Müllerian duct cysts, 158
    Skene gland cysts, 157–158, 158f
    urethral diverticula, 4, 5f, 157, 157f, 158f
  imaging for, 159–160
  nonoperative management, 159
  outcomes, 170–171
  pearls and pitfalls, 170
  postoperative care, 170
  preoperative planning, 160
  procedures and techniques
    Skene gland cyst excision, 167p–168p
    transurethral diverticulotomy or unroofing, 166p
    transvaginal urethral diverticulectomy, 162p–165p
    vaginal wall cyst excision, 169p
  surgical management, 160–161
    approach, 161
    positioning, 161
Urethral incontinence, postrepair, 121–122
Urethrovaginal fistula, 99, 99f, 100, 171
Urge urinary incontinence (UUI), 67. *See also* Urinary incontinence (UI)
Urinalysis, 67
Urinary frequency, 67
Urinary incontinence (UI), 67–96, 143
  complications, 95–96
  definition, 67
  diagnostic evaluation, 69–70
  dietary bladder triggers, 68t
  differential diagnosis, 67
  goal of treatment, 70
  mixed, 67
  nonoperative management, 68–69
    behavior and lifestyle modifications, 68

Urinary incontinence (*continued*)
    dietary intake, 68, 68t
    medical management, 69, 69t
    pelvic floor muscle exercises, 69
    posterior tibial nerve stimulation, 69, 69f
  outcomes, 95
  pearls and pitfalls, 94
  physical examination, 67, 68t
  postoperative care, 95, 95t
  preoperative planning, 70–71
    cystoscopy under local anesthesia, 70
    patients with SUI and, 70–71, 70f, 71f
    patients with UUI and, 71, 71f
  procedures and techniques
    cystoscopic injection with botulinum toxin, 86p–87p
    mid-urethral slings, 73p–80p
    pubovaginal slings, 81p–84p
    sacral neuromodulation, 88p–93p
    transurethral slings, 85p–87p
  stress, 67
  surgical management, 71
    approach, 72
    patient positioning, 71–72, 72f
  urgency, 67
Urine dermatitis, 99, 100f
Urodynamics, 70, 145
Uterine manipulator, 56p
Uterosacral ligaments (USL), 51, 52f
  and cardinal ligament complex, 19, 19f

Uterosacral ligament vault suspension, for apical prolapse, 22p–25p
Uterovaginal fistula, 99, 99f

V

Vaginal foreign body, 5, 5f
Vaginal manipulators, 56p
Vaginal mesh, removal of, 143
  complications, 152–153
  diagnostic evaluation, 144–145, 145f
  differential diagnosis, 144
  general principles, 143–144
  nonoperative management, 144
  outcomes, 153
  pearls and pitfalls, 152
  physical examination, 143–144
  postoperative care, 152
    antibiotics, 152
    continuous bladder drainage, 152
    physical activity restriction, 152
  preoperative planning, 145
    complete excision, 146, 146f
    partial mesh excision and revision, 145–146
  procedures and techniques, 147p
    complete excision, 147p–148p
    incision planning, 147p
    partial excision of mesh, 147p
    retropubic arm removal, 151p
    technique, 149p–150p
    transobturator arm removal, 151p

  surgical management, 146
    approach, 146
    patient positioning, 146
Vaginal prolapse
  anterior (*see* Anterior vaginal wall repair)
  apical (*see* Apical prolapse repair, abdominal approach; Apical prolapse, vaginal repair of)
  posterior (*see* Posterior vaginal wall repair)
Vaginal wall inclusion cyst, 4, 5f
Vagina, nonfunctional, 122
Vaginography, 128
Vascular tissue interposition flaps, 114p
VCUG. *See* Voiding cystourethrography (VCUG)
Vesicovaginal fistula, 99, 99f
  abdominal approach for, 109p
    extravesical approaches, 113p
    O'Conor transperitoneal supravesical technique, 109p–113p
  vaginal approach for, 104p–107p
Voiding cystourethrography (VCUG), 101, 101f, 102f, 145, 159–160
Vulvar urine dermatitis, 99, 100f

W

Wolffian duct cysts. *See* Gartner duct cysts